METHODS IN MOLECULAR BIOLOGY

Series Editor
John M. Walker
School of Life and Medical Sciences
University of Hertfordshire
Hatfield, Hertfordshire, AL10 9AB, UK

For further volumes:
http://www.springer.com/series/7651

Bacterial Therapy of Cancer

Methods and Protocols

Edited by

Robert M. Hoffman

AntiCancer, Inc., University of California San Diego, San Diego, CA, USA

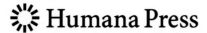 Humana Press

Editor
Robert M. Hoffman
AntiCancer Inc.
University of California San Diego
San Diego, CA, USA

ISSN 1064-3745   ISSN 1940-6029   (electronic)
Methods in Molecular Biology
ISBN 978-1-4939-3513-0   ISBN 978-1-4939-3515-4   (eBook)
DOI 10.1007/978-1-4939-3515-4

Library of Congress Control Number: 2015960794

Springer New York Heidelberg Dordrecht London

Cover Page: Zhao, M., Yang, M., Li, X-M., Jiang, P., Baranov, E., Li, S., Xu, M., Penman, S., and Hoffman, R.M. Tumor-targeting bacterial therapy with amino acid auxotrophs of GFP-expressing *Salmonella typhimurium*. Proc. Natl. Acad. Sci. USA 102, 755–760, 2005.

Printed on acid-free paper

Humana Press is a brand of Springer
Springer Science+Business Media LLC New York is part of Springer Science+Business Media (www.springer.com)

Dedication

This book is dedicated to the memory of A.R. Moossa, M.D., and Sun Lee, M.D.

Introduction

The potential of bacteria to cure cancer has been documented for hundreds of years. In the late nineteenth and early twentieth centuries, bacterial therapy of cancer was first-line at one of the most important cancer hospitals in the world, New York Hospital (later to become the Memorial Sloan Kettering Cancer Center), directed by Dr. William B. Coley, arguably one of the most important oncologists in history. However, Dr. Coley had a great discreditor at his hospital, the renowned pathologist James Ewing, who ended Coley's career and thereby ended bacterial therapy of cancer in the 1930s. However, in modern times, there has been a great revival of bacterial cancer therapy and the exciting chapters of this book chronicle this modern revolution.

Hoffman in the Preface briefly chronicles the long history of bacterial therapy of cancer.

Hoffman in Chapter 1 describes the development of the tumor-targeting *Salmonella typhimurium* A1-R.

Fang et al. in Chapter 2 describe the use of enhanced permeability and retention (EPR) effect by means of nitroglycerin (NG) to enhance the delivery of *Lactobacillus casei* to tumors.

Wei and Jia in Chapter 3 describe the oral delivery of tumor-targeting *Salmonella* for cancer therapy in a mouse tumor model.

Brackett et al. in Chapter 4 describe a microfluidic device for precise quantification of the interactions between tumor-targeting bacteria and tumor tissue.

Taniguchi et al. in Chapter 5 describe methods and protocols for use of the non-pathogenic obligate anaerobic *Bifidobacterium longum* as a drug delivery system (DDS) to target tumor tissues with anaerobic environments.

Leschner and Weiss in Chapter 6 describe noninvasive in vivo imaging of bacteria-mediated cancer therapy using bioluminescent bacteria.

Cronin et al. in Chapter 7 describe the use of whole-body bioluminescence imaging for the study of bacterial trafficking in live mice within tumors following systemic administration.

Lee in Chapter 8 describes attenuated *Salmonella* carrying a eukaryotic expression plasmid encoding an antiangiogenic gene for tumor targeting and gene delivery in murine tumor models and the use of a polymer to shield *Salmonella* from immune responses.

Chiang et al. in Chapter 9 describe targeted delivery of a transgene (eukaryotic GFP) by *Escherichia coli* to HER2/*neu*-positive cancer cells.

Low et al. in Chapter 10 describe deficient *msbB Salmonella* strains that exhibit sensitivities to common metabolites and CO_2 and suppressor mutations that compensate for these sensitivities.

Kramer in Chapter 11 describes facile and precise methods for determining the kinetics of plasmid loss or maintenance in tumor-targeting bacteria.

Nguyen and Min in Chapter 12 describe a method to achieve remote control of therapeutic gene expression in tumor-targeting bacteria.

Hoffman and Zhao in Chapter 13 describe methods for *S. typhimurium* A1-R targeting of primary and metastatic tumors in monotherapy in nude mouse models of major types of human cancer.

Hoffman and Yano describe the cell-cycle decoy of cancer cells resistant to cytotoxic drugs to drug sensitivity by *S. typhimurium* A1-R.

Hoffman describes the future potential of bacterial therapy of cancer.

Robert M. Hoffman

Preface: A Brief History of Bacterial Therapy of Cancer

Anecdotal records go back at least 200 years describing cancer patients going into remission after a bacterial infection [1]. In 1867, the German physician Busch reported that a cancer went into remission when the patient contracted erysipelas, now known as *Streptococcus pyogenes* [2]. Bruns intentionally injected a cancer patient in 1888 with *S. pyogenes* and the tumor regressed [1].

In the late 1890s, William B. Coley of New York Cancer Hospital, later to become Memorial Sloan-Kettering Cancer Center, treated cancer patients with *S. pyogenes*. Coley read about 47 cases of cancer where the patient became infected with bacteria and tumors regressed [3]. Coley located a former patient from his institute whose malignant tumor in his neck regressed after he became infected with erysipelas. When Coley located the patient, he had no evidence of cancer [3]. Coley also found a sarcoma patient in 1891 who had tumor regression also after infection with *S. pyogenes*. Koch, Pasteur, and von Behring recorded that cancer patients infected with *S. pyogenes* had tumor regression [1].

Coley's first patient that he infected with *S. pyogenes* recovered from head and neck cancer. Coley had excellent results infecting cancer patients with *S. pyogenes*. Coley subsequently used killed *S. pyogenes* with a second killed organism now known as *Serratia marcescens*, due to fears of infecting cancer patients with live bacteria. The killed organisms became known as Coley's Toxins. Coley's Toxins are thought to be the beginning of the field of cancer immunology, and many researchers believe that the main anticancer efficacy of bacteria is immunological, but as can be seen in this book, bacteria can directly kill cancer cells as well.

Coley was unfairly criticized by the scientific community and called a quack [3]. During Coley's time, X-rays and surgery became the main treatment of cancer, and their proponents heavily opposed Coley's bacterial therapy, especially James Ewing, a very famous cancer pathologist for whom the Ewing sarcoma is named. Ewing tried to force Coley out of the New York Cancer Hospital, even though Coley had successfully treated hundreds of cancer patients. Ewing was Medical Director of New York Cancer Hospital, therefore Coley's boss, and they hated each other. Ewing would only allow radiation therapy and surgery for all bone tumors, and Ewing did not allow Coley to use his toxins [3]. Coley died deeply disappointed in 1936 and thus ended bacterial therapy of cancer for almost 70 years.

In modern times, Hoption Cann et al. [4] compared Coley's bacterial treatment to current chemotherapy. The 10-year survival rates of Coley's patients were compared to the Surveillance Epidemiology End Result Cancer Registry [5] and found patients receiving current conventional therapies did not fare better than patients treated with bacteria over 100 years ago.

In the middle of the last century, preclinical studies began with bacterial therapy of cancer and are now very widespread. Malmgren and Flanigan [6] demonstrated that anaerobic bacteria could survive and replicate in necrotic tumor tissue with low oxygen content. Several approaches aimed at utilizing bacteria for cancer therapy were described in mice [7–19].

In the modern era, the obligate aerobes *Bifidobacterium* [19] and *Clostridium* [20], which replicate only in necrotic areas of tumors, have been developed for cancer therapy. Anaerobic bacteria cannot grow in viable tumor tissue, which limits their efficacy. Yazawa et al. tested *Bifidobacterium longum* and found it selectively localized in mammary tumors after systemic administration [19] (please *see* Chapter 5). *Clostridium novyi*, without its lethal toxin (*C. novyi* no toxin [NT]), was generated by the John Hopkins group. *C. novyi-NT* spores germinated within necrotic areas of tumors in mice and even killed some viable tumor after intravenous (i.v.) injection. *C. novyi-NT* spores were administered in combination with chemotherapy, resulted in hemorrhagic necrosis and tumor regression [20]. Recently, *C. novyi*-NT was used in a patient with leiomyosarcoma and caused one metastatic lesion to regress [21]. The disadvantage of the obligate anaerobes described above is that they do not grow in viable regions of tumors due to high oxygen tension [2, 22].

Salmonella typhimurium (*S. typhimurium*) is a facultative anaerobe, which can grow in the viable regions as well as necrotic regions of tumors [23]. Attenuated auxotrophic mutants of *S. typhimurium* retained their tumor-targeting capabilities, but became safe to use in mice and humans [24]. *S. typhimurium* with the lipid A–mutation (msbB) deleted and purine auxotrophic mutations (purI) had antitumor efficacy in mice and swine and also had significantly reduced host TNF-a induction and low toxicity. *S. typhimurium* (VNP20009), attenuated by msbB and purI mutations, was safely administered to patients, in a phase I clinical trial on patients with metastatic melanoma and renal carcinoma. Efficacy was not observed, perhaps due to overattenuation [25].

The coming decade should see the resurgence of bacterial therapy of cancer begun by Coley. This book sets the stage for this upcoming revolution of cancer therapy.

After reading this book, one may wonder where cancer therapy would be if Ewing did not so cruelly end Coley's bacterial treatment and eliminate any chance for a successor.

San Diego, CA   *Robert M. Hoffman*

References

1. William Coley. http://en.wikipedia.org/wiki/William_Coley. Accessed 12 Dec 2013
2. Forbes NS (2010) Engineering the perfect (bacterial) cancer therapy. Nat Rev Cancer 10: 785–794
3. McCarthy EF (2006) The toxins of William B. Coley ad the treatment of bone and soft-tissue sarcomas. Iowa Orthop J 26: 154–158
4. Hoption Cann SA, van Netten JP, van Netten C (2003) Dr William Coley and tumour regression: a place in history or in the future. Postgrad Med J 79: 672–680
5. Richardson MA, Ramirez T, Russell NC, et al. (1999) Coley toxins immunotherapy: a retrospective review. Altern Ther Health Med 5: 42–47
6. Malmgren RA, Flanigan CC (1955) Localization of the vegetative form of *Clostridium tetani* in mouse tumors following intravenous spore administration. Cancer Res 15: 473–478
7. Gericke D, Engelbart K (1964) Oncolysis by clostridia. II. Experiments on a tumor spectrum with a variety of clostridia in combination with heavy metal. Cancer Res 24: 217–221
8. Moese JR, Moese G (1964) Oncolysis by clostridia. I. Activity of Clostridium butyricum (M-55) and other nonpathogenic clostridia against the Ehrlich carcinoma. Cancer Res 24: 212–216
9. Thiele EH, Arison RN, Boxer GE (1964) Oncolysis by clostridia. III. Effects of clostridia and chemotherapeutic agents on rodent tumors. Cancer Res 24: 222–233
10. Kohwi Y, Imai K, Tamura Z, Hashimoto Y (1978) Antitumor effect of Bifidobacterium infantis in mice. Gan 69: 613–618
11. Kimura NT, Taniguchi S, Aoki K, Baba T (1980) Selective localization and growth of Bifidobacterium bifidum in mouse tumors following intravenous administration. Cancer Res 40:2061–2068
12. Fox ME, Lemmon MJ, Mauchline ML, Davis TO, Giaccia AJ, Minton NP, et al. (1996) Anaerobic bacteria as a delivery system for cancer gene therapy: in vitro activation of 5-fluorocytosine by genetically engineered clostridia. Gene Ther 3: 173–178
13. Lemmon MJ, Van Zijl P, Fox ME, Mauchline ML, Giaccia AJ, Minton NP, et al. (1997)

Anaerobic bacteria as a gene delivery system that is controlled by the tumor microenvironment. Gene Ther 4: 791–796

14. Brown JM, Giaccia AJ (1998) The unique physiology of solid tumors: opportunities (and problems) for cancer therapy. Cancer Res 58: 1408–1416

15. Low KB, Ittensohn M, Le T, Platt J, Sodi S, Amoss M, et al. (1999) Lipid A mutant Salmonella with suppressed virulence and TNFalpha induction retain tumor-targeting in vivo. Nat Biotechnol 17: 37–41

16. Clairmont C, Lee KC, Pike J, Ittensohn M, Low KB, Pawelek J, et al. (2000) Biodistribution and genetic stability of the novel antitumor agent VNP20009, a genetically modified strain of Salmonella typhimurium. J Infect Dis 181: 1996–2002

17. Sznol M, Lin SL, Bermudes D, Zheng LM, King I (2000) Use of preferentially replicating bacteria for the treatment of cancer. J Clin Invest 105:1027–1030

18. Yazawa K, Fujimori M, Amano J, Kano Y, Taniguchi S (2000) Bifidobacterium longum as a delivery system for cancer gene therapy: selective localization and growth in hypoxic tumors. Cancer Gene Ther 7: 269–274

19. Yazawa K, Fujimori M, Nakamura T, Sasaki T, Amano J, Kano Y, et al. (2001) Bifidobacterium longum as a delivery system for gene therapy of chemically induced rat mammary tumors. Breast Cancer Res Treat 66: 165–170

20. Dang LH, Bettegowda C, Huso DL, et al. (2001) Combination bacteriolytic therapy for the treatment of experimental tumors. Proc Natl Acad Sci USA 98: 15155–15160

21. Roberts NJ, Zhang L, Janku F, Collins A, Bai RY, Staedtke V, et al. (2014) Intratumoral injection of Clostridium novyi-NT spores induces antitumor responses. Sci Transl Med 6: 249ra111

22. Hoffman RM (2012) Bugging tumors. Cancer Disc 2: 588–590

23. Pawelek JM, Low KB, Bermudes D (2003) Bacteria as tumour-targeting vectors. Lancet Oncol 4: 548–556

24. Pawelek JM, Low KB, Bermudes D (1997) Tumor-targeted Salmonella as a novel anticancer vector. Cancer Res 57: 4537–4544

25. Toso JF, Gill VJ, Hwu P, et al. (2002) Phase I study of the intravenous administration of attenuated *Salmonella typhimurium* to patients with metastatic melanoma. J Clin Oncol 20: 142–152

Contents

Contributors

ALI R. AKIN • *Preclinical Imaging, PerkinElmer, Alameda, CA, USA*

DAVID BERMUDES • *Biology Department, California State University Northridge, Northridge, CA, USA; Interdisciplinary Research Institute for the Science (IRIS), California State University Northridge, Northridge, CA, USA*

EMILY L. BRACKETT • *Department of Chemical Engineering, University of Massachusetts—Amherst, Amherst, MA, USA*

CHIH-HSIANG CHANG • *Department of Chemical Engineering, Feng Chia University, Taichung, Taiwan*

YUN-PENG CHAO • *Department of Chemical Engineering, Feng Chia University, Taichung, Taiwan*

CHUNG-JEN CHIANG • *Department of Medical Laboratory Science and Biotechnology, China Medical University, Taichung, Taiwan*

MICHELLE CRONIN • *Cork Cancer Research Center, Biosciences Institute, University College Cork, Cork, Ireland*

JUN FANG • *Research Institute for Drug Delivery System, Sojo University, Kumamoto, Japan; Laboratory of Microbiology and Oncology, Faculty of Pharmaceutical Sciences, Sojo University, Kumamoto, Japan*

NEIL S. FORBES • *Department of Chemical Engineering, University of Massachusetts—Amherst, Amherst, MA, USA*

KEVIN P. FRANCIS • *Preclinical Imaging, PerkinElmer, Alameda, CA, USA*

MINORU FUJIMORI • *Anaeropharma Science Inc., Matsumoto, Japan; Ibaraki Medical Center, Tokyo Medical University, Ibaraki, Japan*

ROBERT M. HOFFMAN • *AntiCancer Inc., Department of Surgery, University of California, San Diego, CA, USA*

LIJUN JIA • *Cancer Institute, Fudan University Shanghai Cancer Center, Shanghai, China*

MING-CHING KAO • *Department of Biological Science and Technology, China Medical University, Taichung, Taiwan*

M. GABRIELA KRAMER • *Department of Biotechnology, Instituto de Higiene, Facultad de Medicina, Universidad de la Republica, Montevideo, Uruguay*

CHE-HSIN LEE • *Department of Microbiology, School of Medicine, China Medical University, Taichung, Taiwan; Department of Biological Sciences, National Sun Yat-sen University, National Sun Yat-sen University, Taiwan*

SARA LESCHNER • *Department of Molecular Immunology, Helmholtz Centre for Infection Research, Braunschweig, Germany*

LIAO LONG • *Research Institute for Drug Delivery System, Sojo University, Kumamoto, Japan*

K. BROOKS LOW • *Department of Therapeutic Radiology, School of Medicine, Yale University, New Haven, CT, USA*

HIROSHI MAEDA • *Research Institute for Drug Delivery System, Sojo University, Kumamoto, Japan; Laboratory of Microbiology and Oncology, Faculty of Pharmaceutical Sciences, Sojo University, Kumamoto, Japan*

JUNG-JOON MIN • *Laboratory of In Vitro Molecular Imaging, Department of Nuclear Medicine, Chonnam National University Medical School, Gwangju, South Korea*

SEAN R. MURRAY • *Biology Department, California State University Northridge, Northridge, CA, USA; Interdisciplinary Research Institute for the Science (IRIS), California State University Northridge, Northridge, CA, USA*

VU H. NGUYEN • *Laboratory of In Vitro Molecular Imaging, Department of Nuclear Medicine, Chonnam National University Medical School, Gwangju, South Korea*

JOHN PAWALEK • *Department of Dermatology, School of Medicine, Yale University, New Haven, CT, USA*

YUKO SHIMATANI • *Anaeropharma Science Inc., Matsumoto, Japan*

CHARLES A. SWOFFORD • *Department of Chemical Engineering, University of Massachusetts—Amherst, Amherst, MA, USA*

MARK TANGNEY • *Cork Cancer Research Center, Biosciences Institute, University College Cork, Cork, Ireland*

SHUN'ICHIRO TANIGUCHI • *Department of Advanced Medicine for Health Promotion, Institute for Biomedical Sciences, Interdisciplinary Cluster for Cutting Edge Research, Shinshu University Graduate School of Medicine, Matsumoto, Japan; Anaeropharma Science Inc., Matsumoto, Japan*

DONGPING WEI • *Cancer Institute, Fudan University Shanghai Cancer, Shanghai, China; Department of Oncology, Nanjing First Hospital, Nanjing Medical University, Nanjing, China*

SIEGFRIED WEISS • *Department of Molecular Immunology, Helmholtz Centre for Infection Research, Braunschweig, Germany*

SHUYA YANO • *AntiCancer Inc. and Department of Surgery, University of California – San Diego, San Diego, CA, USA*

MING ZHAO • *AntiCancer Inc., and Department of Surgery, University of California – San Diego, San Diego, CA, USA*

Chapter 1

Tumor-Targeting *Salmonella typhimurium* A1-R: An Overview

Robert M. Hoffman

Abstract

The present chapter reviews the development of the tumor-targeting amino-acid auxotrophic strain *S. typhimurium* A1 and the in vivo selection and characterization of the high-tumor-targeting strain *S. typhimurium* A1-R. Efficacy of *S. typhimurium* A1-R in nude-mouse models of prostate, breast, pancreatic, and ovarian cancer, as well as sarcoma and glioma in orthotopic mouse models is described. Also reviewed is efficacy of *S. typhimurium A1-R* targeting of primary bone tumor and lung metastasis of high-grade osteosarcoma, breast-cancer brain metastasis, and experimental breast-cancer bone metastasis in orthotopic mouse models. The efficacy of *S. typhimurium* A1-R on pancreatic cancer stem cells, on pancreatic cancer in combination with anti-angiogenic agents, as well as on cervical cancer, soft-tissue sarcoma, and pancreatic cancer patient-derived orthotopic xenograft (PDOX) mouse models, is also described.

Key words Salmonella typhimurium A1-R, Tumor targeting, Amino acid, Auxotroph, Green fluorescent protein (GFP), Cancer-cell killing, Nude mice, Mouse models, Cancer, Metastasis, Orthotopic, Patient-derived orthotopic xenograft (PDOX)

1 Introduction

1.1 Development of Tumor-Targeting Amino-Acid Auxotrophic Strain *S. typhimurium* A1

1. *Green fluorescent protein (GFP) transformation of S. typhimurium.* S. typhimurium 14028 was transfected with the pGFP gene by electroporation. The transformed *S. typhimurium* expressed GFP over 100 passages with GFP expression monitored at each passage [1].

2. *Generation of auxotrophs of S. typhimurium GFP* [1]. *S. typhimurium* auxotrophic strains were obtained with nitroso-guanidine (NTG) mutagenesis. After inoculation with wild-type *S. typhimurium*, the mice died within 2 days. Mutated bacteria were inoculated in mice to see if they survived longer than mice inoculated with wild-type *S. typhimurium*. The mice which lived longest were those inoculated with auxotroph A1

Robert M. Hoffman (ed.), *Bacterial Therapy of Cancer: Methods and Protocols*, Methods in Molecular Biology, vol. 1409, DOI 10.1007/978-1-4939-3515-4_1, © Springer Science+Business Media New York 2016

and they survived as long as control uninfected mice. A1 required Leu and Arg and was chosen for efficacy studies.

3. *Cancer cell killing by S. typhimurium A1* in vitro. PC-3 human prostate cancer cells were labeled with red fluorescent protein (RFP) in the cytoplasm with retroviral RFP and GFP in the nucleus by means of a fusion of GFP with histone H2B. Interaction between bacteria and cancer cells was visualized by dual-color imaging [1].

1.2 Efficacy of S. typhimurium A1 in Nude Mouse Models of Prostate and Breast Cancer

PC-3-RFP human prostate cancer cells were implanted subcutaneously (s.c.) in nude mice. Tumor size was determined from fluorescence imaging at each time point after infection. *S. typhimurium* A1 selectively colonized the PC-3 tumor and strongly suppressed its growth [1].

1.3 In Vivo Selection and Characterization of High-Tumor-Targeting Strain S. typhimurium A1-R

1. To obtain an enhanced tumor-targeting variants, *S. typhimurium* A1 was passaged in nude mice transplanted with the HT-29 human colon tumor. GFP-expressing bacteria were isolated from the infected tumor and were then cultured. The selected *S. typhimurium* A1 was termed *S. typhimurium* A1-R. *S. typhimurium* A1-R attached to HT-29 human colon cancer cells sixfold greater than parental *S. typhimurium* A1 [2].

   In another experiment, *S. typhimurium* A1 and *S. typhimurium* A1-R both infected dual-color PC-3 cancer cells expressing GFP in the nucleus and RFP in the cytoplasm. PC-3 cells which were infected in vitro with *S. typhimurium* A1-R died within 2 h, compared to 24 h *S. typhimurium* A1 infection [3]. *S. typhimurium* A1-R had 100× greater colony forming units (CFU) in PC-3 tumor tissue than *S. typhimurium* A1 [3].

2. *Tumor targeting by S. typhimurium A1-R.* The ratio of *S. typhimurium* A1-R in tumors compared to normal tissue was approximately 10^6, indicating a very high degree of tumor targeting by *S. typhimurium* A1-R [3].

1.4 Efficacy of S. typhimurium A1-R on Prostate Cancer Orthotopic Mouse Models

S. typhimurium A1-R could eradicate tumors in orthotopic nude mouse models of PC-3. Of ten mice with PC-3 tumors that were injected weekly with *S. typhimurium* A1-R, seven were alive at the time the last untreated mouse died. Four of the tumor-bearing mice were apparently cured by weekly bacterial treatment [3].

1.5 Efficacy of S. typhimurium A1-R on Breast Cancer Orthotopic Mouse Models

In orthotopic models of the MARY-X human breast cancer, *S. typhimurium* A1-R led to tumor regression following a single i.v. injection of *S. typhimurium* A1-R [2]. The survival of the *S. typhimurium* A1-R-treated mice with orthotopic MARY-X tumors was prolonged. In some mice, tumors were completely eradicated with no regrowth. The parental *S. typhimurium* A1 was less effective than *S. typhimurium* A1-R [2].

1.6 Efficacy of S. typhimurium A1-R on Pancreatic Cancer Orthotopic Mouse Models

1. *Intracellular growth of S. typhimurium A1-R. S. typhimurium A1-R* invaded and replicated intracellularly in the XPA-1 human pancreatic cancer cell line expressing GFP in the nucleus and RFP in the cytoplasm. Intra-cellular bacterial infection led to cell fragmentation and cell death [4].

2. *Efficacy of S. typhimurium A1-R on an orthotopic pancreatic cancer* in vivo. Tumor growth area was reduced more in the high-bacteria treatment group than the low-bacteria treatment group [4].

3. *Targeting S. typhimurium A1-R to pancreatic cancer liver metastasis.* Mice treated with *S. typhimurium* A1-R intra-splenically (i.s.) or i.v. had a much lower hepatic and splenic tumor burden compared to untreated control mice. i.v. treatment with *S. typhimurium* A1-R also increased survival time [5].

1.7 Efficacy of S. typhimurium A1-R on Glioma Orthotopic Mouse Models

1. U87-RFP human glioma cells were injected stereotactically into the mouse brain. *S. typhimurium* A1-R was administered by injection through a craniotomy open window (i.c.) or i.v. in nude mice 2 weeks after glioma cell implantation. Mice were treated with *S. typhimurium* A1-R, once a week for 3 weeks. Brain tumors were observed by fluorescence imaging through the craniotomy open window over time. *S. typhimurium* A1-R i.c. inhibited brain tumor growth 7.6-fold compared with untreated mice and improved survival 73 % [6].

2. Spinal cord gliomas are highly malignant and often lead to paralysis and death due to their infiltrative nature, high recurrence rate, and limited treatment options. *S. typhimurium* A1-R was administered i.v. or intra-thecally to the spinal cord cancer in orthotopic mouse models. Tumor fragments of U87-RFP were implanted by surgical orthotopic implantation into the dorsal site of the spinal cord. Untreated mice showed progressive paralysis beginning at day 6 after tumor transplantation and developed complete paralysis between 18 and 25 days. Mice treated i.v. with A1-R had onset of paralysis at approximately 11 days and at 30 days, five mice developed complete paralysis, while the other three mice had partial paralysis. Mice treated by intra-thecal injection of A1-R had onset of paralysis at approximately 18 days, and one mouse was still not paralyzed at day 30. Only one mouse developed complete paralysis at day 30 in this group. Intra-thecally-treated animals had a significantly better survival than the i.v.-treated group as well as the control group [7].

1.8 Efficacy of S. typhimurium A1-R on an Ovarian Cancer Orthotopic Mouse Model

Orthotopic and peritoneal-dissemination mouse models of ovarian cancer were made with the human ovarian cancer cell line SKOV-3-GFP. There was a significant difference in tumor size and survival between mice treated with *S. typhimurium* A1-R and untreated mice [8].

Both i.v. and i.p. *S. typhimurium* A1-R treatment effected prolonged survival of mice with peritoneal-disseminated ovarian cancer compared with the untreated control group. However, i.p. treatment was less toxic than i.v. because selective tumor targeting was most effective with i.p. administration [9].

1.9 Efficacy of S. typhimurium A1-R on a Soft-Tissue Sarcoma in an Orthotopic Mouse Model

HT-1080-RFP human fibrosarcoma cells were injected intramuscularly in nude mice. *S. typhimurium* A1-R was administered via the tail vein from day 14, once a week for 2 weeks. Spontaneous lung metastasis was greatly reduced by *S. typhimurium* A1-R. A mouse model of experimental lung metastasis was obtained by tail vein injection of HT-1080-RFP cells. *S. typhimurium* A1-R also significantly reduced lung metastases and improved overall survival in this model [10].

1.10 Targeting Metastasis with S. typhimurium A1-R

1. XPA-1-RFP human pancreatic cancer cells were injected into the inguinal lymph node in nude mice. Just after injection, cancer cells were imaged trafficking in the efferent lymph duct to the axillary lymph node. Metastasis in the axillary-lymph node was subsequently formed. *S. typhimurium* A1-R was then injected into the inguinal lymph node to target the axillary-lymph node metastasis. Just after bacterial injection, a large amount of bacteria were visualized around the axillary lymph node metastasis. By day 7, all lymph-node metastases had been eradicated in the *S. typhimurium* A1-R-treated mice in contrast to growing metastases in the control group [11].

2. HT-1080-GFP-RFP human fibrosarcoma cells were injected into the footpad of nude mice. The presence of popliteal lymph-node metastasis was determined by weekly imaging. Once the metastasis was detected, *S. typhimurium* A1-R was injected subcutaneously in the footpad [11]. The injected bacteria trafficked in the lymphatic channel. A large amount of *S. typhimurium* A1-R-GFP targeted the popliteal lymph-node metastasis. Dual-color labeling of the cancer cells distinguished them from the GFP-expressing bacteria. All lymph-node metastases shrank, and five out of six were eradicated within 7–21 days after treatment, in contrast to growing metastases in the untreated control group.

3. HT1080-RFP-GFP cells were injected into the tail vein of nude mice to obtain experimental lung metastasis. On days 4 and 11, *S. typhimurium* A1-R was injected in the tail vein. The number of metastases on the surface of the lung was significantly lower in the treatment group than in the control group [11].

1.11 Efficacy of S. typhimurium A1-R Targeting of Primary Bone Tumors and Lung Metastasis of High-Grade Osteosarcoma in Orthotopic Mouse Models

Mice were transplanted with 143B-RFP osteosarcoma cells in the tibia and developed primary bone tumors and lung metastasis. *S. typhimurium* A1-R was administered i.v. and was effective for both primary and metastatic osteosarcoma [12].

1.12 Efficacy of S. typhimurium A1-R on Breast-Cancer Brain Metastasis in Orthotopic Mouse Models

High brain-metastatic variants of murine 4T1 breast cancer cells expressing RFP were injected orthotopically in the mammary fat pad in nude mice. The primary tumor was surgically resected in order to allow brain metastasis to develop. The breast-cancer cells that reached the brain extravasated and grew peri-vascularly and intra-vascularly, and some of the cells proliferated within the vasculature. *S. typhimurium* A1-R significantly inhibited brain metastasis and increased survival [13].

1.13 Efficacy of S. typhimurium A1-R on Experimental Breast-Cancer Bone Metastasis Models

Treatment with *S. typhimurium* A1-R completely prevented bone growth of high metastatic variants of human MDA-MB-435 breast cancer cells injected intra-cardially in nude mice. After injection of the high-bone-metastatic breast cancer variant in the tibia of nude mice, *S. typhimurium* A1-R treatment significantly reduced tumor growth in the bone [14].

1.14 S. typhimurium A1-R Targets Tumor Vascularity

RFP-expressing Lewis lung cancer cells (LLC-RFP) were transplanted subcutaneously in the ear, back skin, and footpad of nestin-driven GFP (ND-GFP) transgenic nude mice, which selectively express GFP in nascent blood vessels. Tumor vascularity correlated positively with the anti-tumor efficacy of *S. typhimurium* A1-R. These results suggest that *S. typhimurium* A1-R efficacy on tumors involves vessel destruction which depends on the extent of vascularity of the tumor [15].

Leschner et al. [16] observed a rapid increase of TNF-α in the blood, in addition to other pro-inflammatory cytokines, after *S. typhimurium* treatment of tumors. This induced a great influx of the blood into the tumors by vascular disruption, and bacteria were flushed into the tumor along with the blood [16]. These results also indicated that the degree of vascularity is most important when bacteria target tumors and destroy tumor blood vessels [15].

1.15 Efficacy of S. typhimurium A1-R on Tumors in Immuno-competent Mice

S. typhimurium A1-R was determined on LLC in C57BL/6 immunocompetent mice. Bolus treatment of *S. typhimurium* A1-R was toxic to the immuno-competent host, in contrast to nude mice. Lower-dose weekly doses and metronomic doses were well tolerated by the immuno-competent host and inhibited metastasis formation. Lung metastasis was significantly inhibited by intra-thoracic bacterial administration, without toxicity [17].

1.16 Determining Optimal Route of Administration of S. typhimurium A1-R

The efficacy and safety of three different routes of *S. typhimurium* A1-R administration, oral (p.o.), intra-venous (i.v.), and intra-tumoral (i.t.), in nude mice with orthotopic human breast cancer, were determined. Nude mice with MDA-MB-435 human breast cancer, expressing RFP, were administered *S. typhimurium* A1-R by each of the three routes. Tumor growth was monitored by fluorescence imaging and caliper measurement in two dimensions. *S. typhimurium* A1-R targeted tumors at much higher levels than normal organs after all three routes of administration. The fewest bacteria were detected in normal organs after p.o. administration, which suggested that p.o. administration has the highest safety. The i.v. route had the greatest antitumor efficacy [18].

1.17 Efficacy of S. typhimurium A1-R on Pancreatic Cancer Stem Cells

The XPA-1 human pancreatic cancer cell line is dimorphic, with spindle stem-like cells and round non-stem cells. Stem-like XPA-1 cells were significantly more resistant than non-stem XPA-1 cells to 5-fluorouracil (5-FU) and cisplatinum (CDDP). In contrast, there was no difference between the efficacy of *S. typhimurium* A1-R on stem-like and non-stem XPA-1 cells. In vivo, 5-FU and *S. typhimurium* A1-R significantly reduced the tumor weight of non-stem XPA-1 cells. In contrast, only *S. typhimurium* A1-R significantly reduced tumor weight of stem-like XPA-1 cells. The combination *S. typhimurium* A1-R with 5-FU improved the anti-tumor efficacy compared with 5-FU monotherapy on the stem-like cells [19].

1.18 Efficacy of S. typhimurium A1-R in Combination with Anti-Angiogenic Agents on Orthotopic Pancreatic Cancer Mouse Models

S. typhimurium A1-R treatment was followed with anti-vascular endothelial growth factor (VEGF) therapy on VEGF-positive human pancreatic cancer in an orthotopic nude mouse model of pancreatic cancer. A pancreatic-cancer patient-derived orthotopic xenograft (PDOX) model that was VEGF-positive and an orthotopic VEGF-positive human pancreatic cancer cell line (MiaPaCa-2-GFP) were tested. *S. typhimurium* A1-R significantly reduced tumor weight compared to bevacizumab (BEV)/gemcitabine (GEM) treatment in the PDOX and MiaPaCa-2 models [20].

1.19 Efficacy of S. typhimurium A1-R on a Cervical Cancer PDOX Mouse Model

The efficacy of *S. typhimurium* A1-R in combination with trastuzumab on a PDOX mouse model of HER-2-positive cervical cancer was determined. The relative tumor volume of *S. typhimurium* A1-R + trastuzumab-treated mice was smaller compared to trastuzumab alone and *S. typhimurium* A1-R alone [21].

1.20 Efficacy of S. typhimurium A1-R in a Soft-Tissue Sarcoma Patient Model

A patient-derived nude mouse model of soft-tissue sarcoma growing subcutaneously was established and treated in the following groups: (1) untreated controls, (2) GEM (80 mg/kg, ip, weekly, 3 weeks), (3) Pazopanib (100 mg/kg, orally, daily, 3 weeks), and (4) *Salmonella typhimurium* A1-R (5×10^7 CFU/body, ip, weekly, 3 weeks). The sarcoma was resistant to GEM. Pazopanib tended to reduce the tumor volume compared to the untreated mice, but there was no significant difference. *S. typhimurium* A1-R was the only effective treatment [22].

1.21 Efficacy of S. typhimurium A1-R on a PDOX Model of Pancreatic Cancer

A pancreatic cancer PDOX was transplanted by surgical orthotopic implantation (SOI) in transgenic nude RFP-expressing mice in order that the PDOX stably acquired RFP-expressing stroma for the purpose of imaging the tumor after passage to non-transgenic nude mice. *S. typhimurium* A1-R treatment significantly reduced tumor weight, as well as tumor fluorescent area, compared to untreated control, with comparable efficacy of GEM, CDDP, and 5-FU [23].

These results demonstrate the therapeutic potential *of S. typhimurium* A1-R on major cancer types, including recalcitrant cancers, such as pancreatic and sarcoma, and justify clinical trials as soon as possible.

References

1. Zhao M, Yang M, Li X-M, Jiang P, Baranov E, Li S et al (2005) Tumor-targeting bacterial therapy with amino acid auxotrophs of GFP-expressing *Salmonella typhimurium*. Proc Natl Acad Sci U S A 102:755–760

2. Zhao M, Yang M, Ma H, Li X, Tan X, Li S et al (2006) Targeted therapy with a *Salmonella typhimurium* leucine-arginine auxotroph cures orthotopic human breast tumors in nude mice. Cancer Res 66:7647–7652

3. Zhao M, Geller J, Ma H, Yang M, Penman S, Hoffman RM (2007) Monotherapy with a tumor-targeting mutant of *Salmonella typhimurium* cures orthotopic metastatic mouse models of human prostate cancer. Proc Natl Acad Sci U S A 104:10170–10174

4. Nagakura C, Hayashi K, Zhao M, Yamauchi K, Yamamoto N, Tsuchiya H et al (2009) Efficacy of a genetically-modified *Salmonella typhimurium* in an orthotopic human pancreatic cancer in nude mice. Anticancer Res 29:1873–1878

5. Yam C, Zhao M, Hayashi K, Ma H, Kishimoto H, McElroy M et al (2010) Monotherapy with a tumor-targeting mutant of *S. typhimurium* inhibits liver metastasis in a mouse model of pancreatic cancer. J Surg Res 164:248–255

6. Momiyama M, Zhao M, Kimura H, Tran B, Chishima T, Bouvet M et al (2012) Inhibition and eradication of human glioma with tumor-targeting *Salmonella typhimurium* in an orthotopic nude-mouse model. Cell Cycle 11:628–632

7. Kimura H, Zhang L, Zhao M, Hayashi K, Tsuchiya H, Tomita K et al (2010) Targeted therapy of spinal cord glioma with a genetically-modified *Salmonella typhimurium*. Cell Prolif 43:41–48

8. Matsumoto Y, Miwa S, Zhang Y, Hiroshima Y, Yano S, Uehara F et al (2014) Efficacy of tumor-targeting *Salmonella typhimurium* A1-R on nude mouse models of metastatic and disseminated human ovarian cancer. J Cell Biochem 115:1996–2003

9. Matsumoto Y, Miwa S, Zhang Y, Zhao M, Yano S, Uehara F et al (2015) Intraperitoneal administration of tumor-targeting *Salmonella typhimurium* A1-R inhibits disseminated human ovarian cancer and extends survival in nude mice. Oncotarget 6:11369–11377

10. Miwa S, Zhang Y, Baek K-E, Uehara F, Yano S, Yamamoto M et al (2014) Inhibition of spontaneous and experimental lung metastasis of soft-tissue sarcoma by tumor-targeting *Salmonella typhimurium* A1-R. Oncotarget 5:12849–12861

11. Hayashi K, Zhao M, Yamauchi K, Yamamoto N, Tsuchiya H, Tomita K et al (2009) Cancer metastasis directly eradicated by targeted therapy with a modified *Salmonella typhimurium*. J Cell Biochem 106:992–998

12. Hayashi K, Zhao M, Yamauchi K, Yamamoto N, Tsuchiya H, Tomita K et al (2009) Systemic targeting of primary bone tumor and lung metastasis of high-grade osteosarcoma in nude mice with a tumor-selective strain of *Salmonella typhimurium*. Cell Cycle 8:870–875

13. Zhang Y, Miwa S, Zhang N, Hoffman RM, Zhao M (2015) Tumor-targeting *Salmonella*

typhimurium A1-R arrests growth of breast-cancer brain metastasis. Oncotarget 6:2615–2622

14. Miwa S, Yano S, Zhang Y, Matsumoto Y, Uehara F, Yamamoto M et al (2014) Tumor-targeting *Salmonella typhimurium* A1-R prevents experimental human breast cancer bone metastasis in nude mice. Oncotarget 5: 7119–7125

15. Liu F, Zhang L, Hoffman RM, Zhao M (2010) Vessel destruction by tumor-targeting Salmonella typhimurium A1-R is enhanced by high tumor vascularity. Cell Cycle 9:4518–4524

16. Leschner S, Westphal K, Dietrich N, Viegas N, Jablonska J, Lyszkiewicz M et al (2009) Tumor invasion of Salmonella enterica serovar Typhimurium is accompanied by strong hemorrhage promoted by TNF-a. PLoS One 4:e6692

17. Zhao M, Suetsugu A, Ma H, Zhang L, Liu F, Zhang Y et al (2012) Efficacy against lung metastasis with a tumor-targeting mutant of *Salmonella typhimurium* in immunocompetent mice. Cell Cycle 11:187–193

18. Zhang Y, Tome Y, Suetsugu A, Zhang L, Zhang N, Hoffman RM et al (2012) Determination of the optimal route of administration of *Salmonella typhimurium* A1-R to target breast cancer in nude mice. Anticancer Res 32:2501–2508

19. Hiroshima Y, Zhao M, Zhang Y, Maawy A, Hassanein MK, Uehara F et al (2013) Comparison of efficacy of *Salmonella typhimurium* A1-R and chemotherapy on stem-like and non-stem human pancreatic cancer cells. Cell Cycle 12:2774–2780

20. Hiroshima Y, Zhang Y, Murakami T, Maawy AA, Miwa S, Yamamoto M et al (2014) Efficacy of tumor-targeting *Salmonella typhimurium* A1-R in combination with anti-angiogenesis therapy on a pancreatic cancer patient-derived orthotopic xenograph (PDOX) and cell line mouse models. Oncotarget 5:12346–12357

21. Hiroshima Y, Zhang Y, Zhao M, Zhang N, Murakami T, Maawy A et al (2015) Tumor-targeting *Salmonella typhimurium* A1-R in combination with Trastuzumab eradicates HER-2-positive cervical cancer cells in patient-derived mouse models. PLoS One 10:e0120358

22. Hiroshima Y, Zhao M, Zhang Y, Zhang N, Maawy A, Murakami T et al (2015) Tumor-targeting *Salmonella typhimurium* A1-R arrests a chemo-resistant patient soft-tissue sarcoma in nude mice. PLoS One 10:e0134324

23. Hiroshima Y, Zhao M, Maawy A, Zhang Y, Katz MH, Fleming JB et al (2014) Efficacy of *Salmonella typhimurium* A1-R versus chemotherapy on a pancreatic cancer patient-derived orthotopic xenograft (PDOX). J Cell Biochem 115:1254–1261

Chapter 2

Enhancement of Tumor-Targeted Delivery of Bacteria with Nitroglycerin Involving Augmentation of the EPR Effect

Jun Fang, Liao Long, and Hiroshi Maeda

Abstract

The use of bacteria, about 1 μm in size, is now becoming an attractive strategy for cancer treatment. Solid tumors exhibit the enhanced permeability and retention (EPR) effect for biocompatible macromolecules such as polymer-conjugated anticancer agents, liposomes, and micelles. This phenomenon permits tumor-selective delivery of such macromolecules. We report here that bacteria injected intravenously evidenced a property similar to that can of these macromolecules. Bacteria that can accumulate selectively in tumors may therefore be used in cancer treatment.

Facultative or anaerobic bacteria will grow even under the hypoxic conditions present in solid tumors. We found earlier that nitric oxide (NO) was among the most important factors that facilitated the EPR effect via vasodilatation, opening of endothelial cell junction gaps, and increasing the blood flow of hypovascular tumors. Here, we describe the augmentation of the EPR effect by means of nitroglycerin (NG), a commonly used NO donor, using various macromolecular agents in different tumor models. More importantly, we report that NG significantly enhanced the delivery of *Lactobacillus casei* to tumors after intravenous injection of the bacteria, more than a tenfold increase in bacterial accumulation in tumors after NG treatment. This finding suggests that NG has a potential advantage to enhance bacterial therapy of cancer, and further investigations of this possibility are warranted.

Key words EPR effect, Nitroglycerin, Nitric oxide, *Lactobacillus casei*, Macromolecules, Solid tumors

1 Introduction

Extravasation of biocompatible macromolecules including polymer–drug conjugates, micelles, and liposomes as well as bacteria about 1 μm in size is observed in most solid tumor tissues. This phenomenon was named the enhanced permeability and retention (EPR) effect of macromolecules in solid tumors [1]. The EPR effect is becoming a gold standard in the design of macromolecular anticancer drugs and tumor-targeted drug delivery systems [2]. The EPR effect is now known to play a major role in tumor-selective delivery of macromolecular drugs, so-called nanomedicines [2–5].

Robert M. Hoffman (ed.), *Bacterial Therapy of Cancer: Methods and Protocols*, Methods in Molecular Biology, vol. 1409, DOI 10.1007/978-1-4939-3515-4_2, © Springer Science+Business Media New York 2016

In experimental tumor models, nanomedicines had 5–100 times greater intra-tumoral drug delivery compared with delivery of the drugs to the blood or normal tissues [4, 5]. Nanomedicines with a molecular weight greater than 50 kDa commonly exhibit the EPR effect, but the effects of molecular weight higher than 800 kDa are poorly understood. Kimura et al. [6] and Hoffman et al. [7], however, reported that some bacteria are preferentially taken up in solid tumors, even bacteria injected intravenously (i.v.).

Anaerobic or facultative bacteria have been known for decades to grow selectively in tumors [6–20]. This growth is now attributed to the unique patho-physiological feature found in many tumors, i.e., impaired and abnormal vascular architecture. Consequently, tumor tissues have high vascular permeability (the EPR effect) and hypoxia, or low pO_2, together with extensive necrosis [5, 7, 18, 20]. In addition, vascular mediators such as nitric oxide (NO) are produced in excess [3–5].

A new anticancer strategy using bacteria was developed and is growing as an attractive option. Hoffman et al. [7, 18] reported that systemic infusion of a modified strain of *Salmonella typhimurium* selectively infected tumor tissues and resulted in significant tumor shrinkage in many tumor (xenograft) models in mice. Taniguchi's group developed tumor-targeted delivery of a prodrug by using genetically engineered *Bifidobacterium longum* expressing cytosine deaminase that would enable the tumor to generate 5-fluorouracil, with remarkable antitumor effects [20]. Both of these methods are now in clinical trials.

Also, Xiang et al. successfully utilized *Escherichia coli* or *Salmonella enterica* serovar typhimurium as a tumor-targeted delivery system to introduce short hairpin RNA into tumor cells that can exhibit RNA interference [19].

In addition, many reports have indicated the anti-tumor therapeutic potential of *Lactobacillus casei*, a non-pathogenic bacterium widely used in dairy products that has enhanced the cellular immunity of the host [21–23]. All these results suggest that bacterial therapy is a promising approach in cancer treatment, and thus, as described in this chapter, the augmentation of bacterial tumor delivery is of great importance.

That the EPR effect is mediated by NO and many other vascular mediators including bradykinin, prostaglandins, and vascular endothelial growth factor is important, and modulating these factors to enhance the EPR effect and achieve tumor-targeted delivery of drugs or bacteria will be critical [5, 24–26]. Among these factors, NO is one of the most important molecules having a vasodilating effect and facilitates increased blood flow as well as increases vascular permeability where it is generated, particularly in tumor tissues [24–26]. As an NO donor, nitroglycerin (NG) has been used for more than a century as a medication, applied topically or orally, for angina pectoris. That NO is generated more in diseased

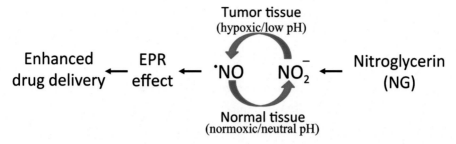

Fig. 1 Hypothetical mechanism of nitric oxide (NO) generation. NO was produced from nitrite, mainly in hypoxic tumor tissues instead of normal tissues. *EPR,* enhanced permeability and retention (from Ref. 30 with permission from the Japanese Cancer Association)

hypoxic tissues, via conversion of nitrite, is of great interest [27–31]. We previously demonstrated that NG was converted to NO in tumor tissues, which exist in a hypoxic state, by mechanisms similar to those operating in infarcted cardiac tissues [28–31]. NG may thus be an ideal NO donor for hypoxic tumors. Figure 1 shows the theoretical mechanism of NO generation from nitrite in tumor tissues and in infarcted cardiac tissues, given that both tissues are similarly hypoxic and acidic.

In view of these data, we previously developed the therapeutic strategy of using topical application of small doses of NG, particularly in combination with macromolecular anti-cancer drugs [30, 31]. More recently, we found that bacteria given by i.v. injection also exhibited enhanced tumor-targeted delivery to a significant extent and with much less delivery of bacteria to normal tissues and organs.

2 Materials

NG ointment (Vasolator®, Sanwa Kagaku Kenkyusho, Nagoya, Japan).

Evans blue dye (Wako Pure Chemical Industries, Osaka, Japan).

7,12-Dimethylbenz[*a*]anthracene (DMBA) (Wako Pure Chemical Industries, Osaka, Japan).

Corn oil (Wako Pure Chemical Industries).

Protoporphyrin IX (Sigma-Aldrich, St. Louis, MO, USA).

Succinimidyl derivative of polyethylene glycol (PEG) (NOF Inc., Tokyo, Japan).

L. casei strain Shirota (Yakult Honsha Co., Ltd., Tokyo, Japan).

MRS (de Man, Rogosa, Sharpe) medium (Cica; Kanto Chemical Co. Inc., Tokyo, Japan).

Lactulose (4-O-β-D-galactopyranosyl-D-fructofuranose) (Wako Pure Chemical Industries).

Female Sprague–Dawley rats (5 weeks old) (SLC, Shizuoka, Japan).

Male ddY mice (6 weeks old) (SLC).

Female BALB/c mice (6 weeks old) (SLC).

Male C57BL/6 J mice (6 weeks old) (SLC).

Mouse S-180 sarcoma cells (2×10^6).

Mouse fibrosarcoma Meth-A cells (2×10^6).

Colon adenocarcinoma C38 cells (2×10^6) (Riken Cell Bank, Tsukuba, Japan).

3   Methods

3.1   Delivery of a Putative Macromolecular Drug (Evans Blue/Albumin Complex) in Combination with NG to Rodent Tumors

When the diameters of S-180 tumors (*see* **Notes 1** and **2**) reached 5–8 mm, NG (*see* **Note 3**) was applied as an ointment to the skin overlying the tumors at doses of 0.001–1.0 mg/tumor, or to normal skin. Within 5 min, 10 mg/kg Evans blue (*see* **Note 4**) in 0.1 mL PBS was injected i.v. At scheduled times thereafter, mice were killed, tumors and normal tissues were removed, weighed, and immersed in 3 mL of formamide followed by incubation at 60 °C for 48 h in order to extract the dye (Evans blue). The concentration of the dye in each tissue was determined spectrophotometrically at 620 nm. Controls in all experiments consisted of treatment with ointment without NG. Similar experiments were carried out in Meth-A, C26 and C38 tumor models (*see* **Notes 1** and **2**) in mice as well as in the DMBA-induced breast tumor model in rats (*see* **Note 2**).

Results showed a time-dependent increase in accumulation of Evans blue/albumin complex in S-180 solid tumors (Fig. 2a, $P=0.006$). NG induced two- to threefold greater drug delivery to solid tumors at 4 h after drug injection than treatment without NG (Fig. 2a, $P=0.002$). Also, tumors retained the higher drug concentration for at least 24 h after NG treatment. Similar results were observed with other solid tumors (Meth-A, C38, and DMBA-induced breast cancer) (Fig. 2c, d). In addition, all tumor models showed NG dose-dependent increases in drug delivery (the EPR effect) (Fig. 2b–d). The effective NG doses were as low as 0.001 mg/tumor up to 2 mg/tumor.

3.2   Macromolecular Drug Delivery to Solid Tumors as Measured by Radioactivity of ^{65}Zn-labeled PZP

NG ointment at 0.1 mg/tumor was applied to the skin by rubbing over S-180 tumors or to non-tumorous abdominal skin, with the distance to tumors of about 5 cm, after which mice immediately received an i.v. injection of ^{65}Zn-labeled PZP (*see* **Note 5**) via the tail vein (12,000 cpm/mouse). After 4 and 24 h, mice were killed and the blood was collected from the inferior vena cava. Mice were then perfused with 10 mL saline containing 5 U/mL heparin to

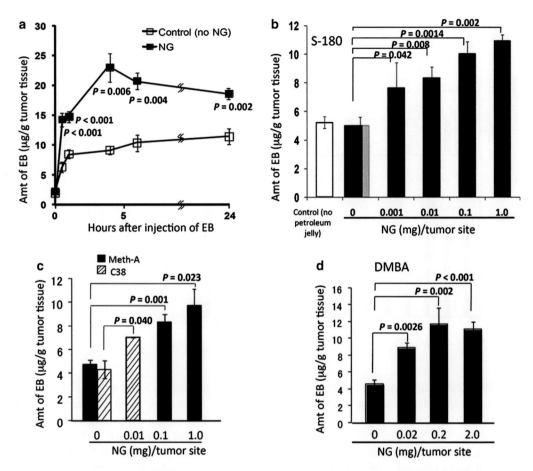

Fig. 2 Time-dependent and nitroglycerin (NG) dose-dependent enhancement of macromolecular drug delivery to solid tumors. (**a**) Time course of enhanced delivery of Evans blue (EB) to S-180 solid tumors by NG ointment (1 mg/tumor) applied to the skin overlying tumors. (**b–d**) Dose-dependent enhancement of delivery of the macromolecular drug to S-180, Meth-A, C38, and 7,12-dimethylbenz[*a*]anthracene (DMBA)-induced breast tumors, respectively. In all models, at tumor diameters of 5–8 mm, 10 mg/kg Evans blue in 0.1 mL PBS was injected intravenously; 4 h later the Evans blue concentration in tumors was quantified. Error bars indicate 95 % confidence intervals. Differences between control (no NG) and NG groups were compared with the Student's *t*-test. Statistical tests were two sided. (from Ref. 30 with permission from the Japanese Cancer Association)

remove blood components from the blood vessels in various organs and tissues. Tumor tissues and normal organs and tissues, including the liver, spleen, kidney, intestine, stomach, colon, heart, brain, lung, skin, muscle, and bone marrow, were collected and weighed. Radioactivity of the samples was measured by using a gamma counter (1480 Wizard 3″; PerkinElmer Life Sciences, Boston, MA, USA).

Similar to the findings with Evans blue as shown in Fig. 2, NG application resulted in about twice the accumulation of PZP in tumors than did ointment without NG, at both 4 and 24 h after drug injection (Fig. 3a, b). This result was also found when NG was applied to the skin at a distance of 5 cm from the tumor (Fig. 3c).

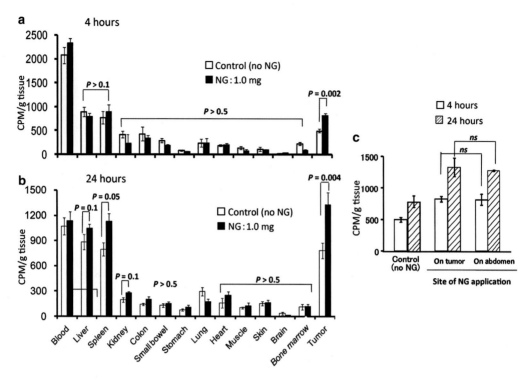

Fig. 3 Nitroglycerin (NG)-enhanced delivery of a radioactive polymeric drug to S-180 solid tumors. NG, in an ointment, was applied to tumor-bearing mice at a dose of 1.0 mg/tumor either to the skin overlying tumors (**a**, **b**) or to non-tumorous dorsal abdominal skin, on the opposite side of the tumor (the distance to the tumor was about 5 cm) (**c**). ^{65}Zn-labeled PZP (12,000 cpm/mouse) was injected intravenously via the tail vein into these mice. After 4 h (**a**) and 24 h (**b**), mice were killed, after which samples of the blood, tumor, and normal tissues and organs were collected, and the radioactivity of these tissues and organs was measured. Error bars show 95 % confidence intervals. Differences between control (no NG) and NG groups were compared with the Student's t-test. Statistical tests were two sided. *CPM*, counts per minute; *ns*, not significant. (from Ref. 30 with permission from the Japanese Cancer Association)

The enhancement of the EPR effect by NG for delivery of macromolecular drugs to tumors was significant ($P=0.002$ and 0.004 at 4 and 24 h, respectively), but findings for most normal organs were not significant, except at 24 h in the spleen and liver ($P=0.05$ and 0.1), which evidenced 15–30 % increased delivery (Fig. 3a, b). Another interesting and important finding was that application of NG to abdominal skin—while the tumor was located on the dorsal skin—produced significantly increased delivery of PZP to the tumor (Fig. 3b, c) but no significant changes in most normal tissues, which suggests that production of NO from NG is tumor-specific, probably because of the hypoxic environment.

3.3 Tumor-Targeted Delivery of L. casei and Its Augmentation by NG

3.3.1 Culture and Quantification of Growth of L. casei

L. casei (see Note 6) was first cultured in MRS agar medium in an agar plate—10 cm (Φ) plastic Petri dish. After 24 h culture at 37 °C, one loop of bacteria, taken from a colony on the agar plate, was placed for additional culture into 10 mL of MRS liquid medium in a 50-mL flask incubated in a water bath at 37 °C with shaking (120 rpm). After overnight incubation, 10 µL of cultured liquid containing the bacteria was transferred into 100 mL of MRS medium in a 300-mL flask, and cultured under the same conditions (37 °C water bath with shaking). The optical density of the cultured bacteria at 600 nm was measured every 30 min. A 10-µL aliquot of the culture was plated on an agar plate followed by incubation at 37 °C to obtain CFU counts after 2 days of incubation. The counts were correlated with optical density.

3.3.2 Pharmacokinetics and Body Distribution of L. casei in ddY Mice Bearing S-180 Solid Tumors With and Without NG Treatment

To investigate the bio-distribution of *L. casei*, 0.1-mL samples (7×10^6 CFU) of bacterial culture were injected via the tail vein, followed by i.p. injection of 1 mL of 20 % lactulose [6]. For the NG-treated group, NG ointment at 0.6 mg/tumor was applied by rubbing over the skin just before the injection of bacteria. At scheduled times (1 and 6 h) after the injection of bacteria, mice were killed and the blood was collected from the inferior vena cava, and mice were then perfused with 10 mL saline containing 5 U/mL heparin to remove blood components from the blood vessels of various organs and tissues. Tumor tissues and normal organs and tissues, including the liver, spleen, kidney, heart, and lung, were collected and weighed. To 1 g of each tissue, 9 mL of cold physiological saline were added, and then tissues were minced and homogenized on ice with a Polytron homogenizer (Kinematica, Littau-Lucerne, Switzerland). Tissue homogenates (50 µL) at different dilutions (10–10,000, obtained by using physiological saline) were transferred to 10-cm petri dishes. Then 15 mL of MRS agar medium, kept at 40 °C in a water bath, was added and thoroughly mixed. The dishes were then placed at room temperature to solidify the agar medium, after which they were placed in an incubator at 37 °C. After 2 days incubation, *L. casei* colonies were counted. The distribution of bacteria in each tissue was expressed as CFU/g tissue or CFU/mL blood.

The results provided in Fig. 4 were similar to those for the putative macromolecular drug (Evans blue/albumin complex, Fig. 2) and the polymeric drug (PZP, Fig. 3). At 1 h after i.v. injection of bacteria, the distribution was noted mostly in the liver and spleen (Fig. 4a). At 6 h, however, the number of bacteria in the liver and spleen decreased markedly to about 1/10 of those at 1 h, whereas the numbers of bacteria in the tumor increased, approximately 80 -fold (Fig. 4b). These findings suggested that bacterial uptake by tumor tissues was due to an EPR effect that was a time-dependent phenomenon, requiring more than several hours (e.g., >4 h in mice; *see* Refs. 4, 31). Moreover, the lower number of bacteria in

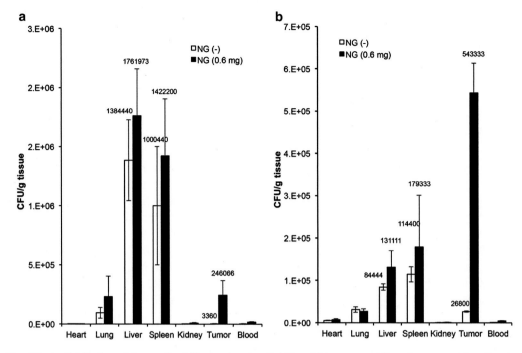

Fig. 4 Body distribution of *L. casei* in ddY mice bearing S-180 solid tumors and its enhancement by nitroglycerin (NG). (**a**) Results at 1 h after i.v. injection of bacteria. (**b**) Results at 6 h after i.v. injection of bacteria. Data are means ± SD. See text for details

the liver and spleen may indicate clearance by the lymphatic and reticuloendothelial systems. Another possibility is that under the hypoxic conditions in tumor tissues, facultative and anaerobic bacteria can grow. More important, normal tissues evidenced no significant uptake of bacteria except for the liver and spleen, in which the reticuloendothelial system is responsible for this function.

Furthermore, NG treatment led to a significant increase in the delivery of bacteria to tumor tissues: approximately 70-fold and 20-fold increases were found at 1 h and 6 h, respectively, after NG treatment (Fig. 4). However, normal tissues including the liver and spleen showed no significant increases (Fig. 4), which suggests that NG was converted to NO predominantly in tumor tissues.

4   Results

4.1   The EPR Effect and Drug Delivery

The EPR effect is considered to be one of the greatest breakthroughs leading to universal targeting to solid tumors in chemotherapy [2, 5, 26, 32]. Matsumura and Maeda first reported the EPR effect in 1986 [1], and Maeda and colleagues continued to perform extensive studies of the effect [3–5, 26]. The EPR effect is based on the fact that most solid tumors have blood vessels with defective architecture and produce excessive amounts of vascular permeability factors. Such enhanced vascular permeability ensures a sufficient supply of nutrients and oxygen to tumor cells to sustain their rapid growth. This unique anatomical–patho-physiological nature of tumor blood vessels was thus utilized to facilitate delivery of macromolecular drugs to tumor tissues. EPR effect-driven drug delivery does not occur in normal tissues, because their vascular architecture manifests tight endothelial junctions and vessels do not produce excess amount of physiological mediators [3–5, 26]. The EPR effect is thus believed to be a landmark principle in tumor-targeting chemotherapy and is becoming a promising paradigm in anticancer drug development [2].

4.2 Macromolecular Drug Delivery to Tumors Based on the EPR Effect

The first macromolecular anticancer drug SMANCS (styrene–maleic acid copolymer-conjugated neocarzinostatin) was approved in Japan for use against liver cancer in 1993. Doxil, which is a PEGylated (PEG-coated) liposome-encapsulated formulation of doxorubicin, is now used in clinical settings to treat Kaposi sarcoma and other cancers. Many other polymeric or micellar drugs are undergoing clinical development (phases I and II) [33, 34]. Compared with conventional small-molecular-mass anti-cancer drugs, macromolecular drugs demonstrate superior in vivo pharmacokinetics (e.g., a prolonged plasma half-life) as well as selective tumor-targeting, which result in improved anti-tumor efficacy with fewer adverse side effects [33, 34].

The EPR effect is a molecular size-dependent phenomenon: biocompatible molecules or particles larger than 50 kDa, which is a limit size for renal clearance, had a prolonged circulation time and very slow renal clearance rate. During circulation, they gradually extravasated from tumor blood vessels and were retained in the tumor tissue for a relatively long time (e.g., several days to weeks) [1, 3–5, 26]. The EPR effect was observed with proteins, polymer conjugates, micelles, liposomes, nanoparticles, DNA polyplexes, lipid particles, and bacteria [1, 3–7, 19–21, 26, 33–35].

Using bacteria is now becoming a promising anti-cancer strategy. Here we confirm the advantage of using bacteria for anticancer therapy based on the EPR effect. After achieving tumor delivery of bacteria, a number of effective mechanisms are then proposed effective for bacterial therapy, for example, utilization of genetically-engineered bacterial toxins or prodrug-activating enzymes or activation of innate immunity including natural killer (NK) cells or other immune cells [6, 7, 18–20, 36–39].

The EPR effect involves vascular heterogeneity, i.e., blood vessels in tumors are not usually evenly distributed, which is observed in most large solid tumors having both hyper- and hypo-vascular areas. Some tumors such as pancreatic and prostate cancer, are hypo-vascular. Because the EPR effect is related to vascular patho-physiology, targeted drug delivery to these hypovascular tumors/areas may be difficult. Methods to augment the EPR effect (blood flow and vascular permeability), especially for hypovascular tumors, are thus important.

4.3 Enhanced Delivery of Macromolecular Drugs and Bacteria to Solid Tumors by NG

As noted above, many vascular mediators are involved in the EPR effect [4, 5, 26]. We have investigated one of these mediators, NO, which is a vital molecule in mammals and has multiple functions such as signal transduction, vasodilatation, increasing the permeability of blood vessels, antioxidant effects, and cell proliferation [5, 39]. In this context, we focused on NG, a well-known NO donor that has been used for more than a century as a medication for angina pectoris. In infarcted-cardiac tissue, NO_2^- is first liberated from NG and is then converted to NO by nitrite reductase under hypoxic conditions (Fig. 1) [27–29]. Vasodilatation and increased blood flow can normalize the blood flow of infarcted tissues. The pO_2 in infarcted-cardiac tissue is low, and the pH is slightly acidic [40, 41], similar to conditions in many tumor tissues. We thus hypothesized that the same situation would occur in tumor tissues as in infarcted-cardiac tissues (Fig. 1; Refs. 26, 31). Application of NG should therefore improve macromolecular drug delivery to tumors having a poor EPR effect, as well as improve the therapeutic efficacy of these drugs.

As expected, we obtained spectacular results in various rodent tumor models, using an Evans blue/albumin complex, polymer conjugates (Figs. 2 and 3; Refs. 26, 29, 31), and bacteria (Fig. 4). These results are similar to those for isosorbide dinitrate [41]. Our results suggested that NG is a useful tool to enhance tumor blood flow, vascular permeability, and the EPR effect to improve tumor-targeted delivery of anti-cancer agents including bacteria.

That NG, in addition to enhancing drug delivery, has a tumor-suppressive effect by itself. NG probably acts by down-regulating the expression of certain critical genes involved in tumor growth [30]. Mitchell et al. [42] and Yasuda et al. [43] also reported that NG increased tumor sensitivity to chemotherapeutic drugs by increasing the blood flow of hypoxic tumors, by suppressing hypoxia-inducible factor-1α, vascular endothelial growth factor, and P-glycoprotein expression in tumors, all of which play important roles in the resistance of cancer cells to such drugs. Combination therapy with NG may therefore produce a significantly additive chemotherapeutic effect by multiple mechanisms, including enhancement of the EPR effect.

Factors and methods other than NG and NO have been investigated to enhance the EPR effect. These methods included angiotensin II-induced hypertension during arterial infusion of SMANCS in cancer patients [4, 5, 44], and the use of angiotensin-converting enzyme inhibitor [26] and the prostacyclin PGI_2 agonist beraprost [45]. We recently found that carbon monoxide (CO), a gas molecule with physiological functions similar to those of NO, also enhanced the EPR effect [46]. Administration of a CO-releasing molecule or its polymer micelles significantly increased extravasation and the accumulation of macromolecular agents in tumors [46].

4.4 L. casei: A Promising Candidate for Bacterial Therapy

L. casei is a nonpathogenic facultatively-anaerobic bacterium that is also a component of the normal bacterial flora in the human intestinal tract and reproductive system. *L. casei* is widely used in various dairy and food supplements, as a so-called probiotic. More important, this bacterium also showed antitumor activity by stimulating nonspecific immune responses, such as macrophage and NK cell activation [36–39], and is considered useful as a medication to prevent recurrence of bladder cancer [21, 22, 47, 48], with mechanisms similar to those of Bacille Calmette-Guérin (BCG) [49]. *L. casei* is thus suitable for bacterial therapy either as a drug vector to carry or deliver genes or as a nonspecific immunostimulant.

With regard to delivery of *L. casei* to tumors, we found tumor-selective accumulation and/or growth of the bacteria after i.v. injection (Fig. 4), which is a result similar to that found in other experiments [6, 7, 18–20]. We now believe that this tumor-preferred accumulation is based on the EPR effect, as discussed above. Moreover, systemic (i.v.) application of the bacteria did not lead to sustained accumulation of bacteria in normal tissues. Although bacteria accumulated mostly in the liver and spleen at 1 h after i.v. injection, the number of *L. casei* decreased dramatically after 6 h (Fig. 4); and at 24 h, almost no bacteria could be found in liver and spleen (Fig. 5). However, the number of bacteria in tumor tissue was far greater than in the liver and spleen (Fig. 5). EPR-based tumor selectivity can induce tumor-specific immune activation and have an anti-tumor effect, with i.v. injection of the bacteria, but not with topical application, such as how BCG for bladder cancer is used. Also, high tumor selectivity will ensure fewer side effects in normal tissues and organs.

More important, as with other macromolecular drugs, NG enhanced the accumulation of bacteria in tumors, i.e., a 70-fold increase at 1 h, 20-fold increase at 6 h and 10-fold increase at 24 h

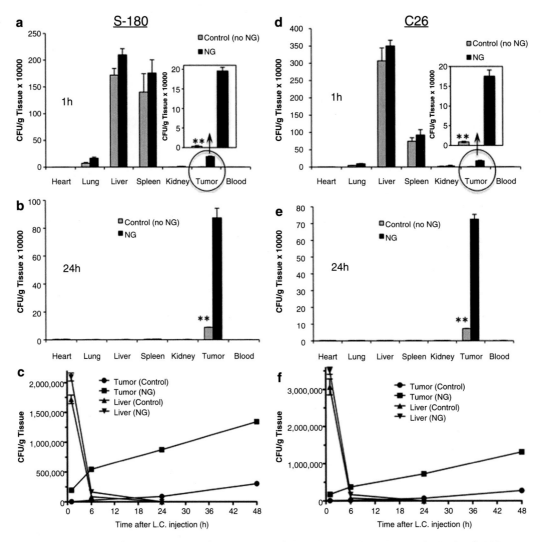

Fig. 5 Enhancement of tumor delivery of L. *casei* by NG. Panels **a–c** show the results in the S-180 tumor model, and **d–f** shows the C26 tumor model. In (**a**) and (**d**), the *insets* show enlarged scales for tumor. In (**c**) and (**f**), time course of accumulation of *L. casei* in tumor and liver with/without NG treatment is shown. Data are means ± SD; $n=6$. **$P<0.01$ (no NG control vs. NG treatment group) (from Ref. [50] with permission)

after i.v. injection of *L. casei* (Figs. 4 and 5). Bacterial therapy may thus be improved by combination with NG and/or other EPR-enhancing agents, and this possibility warrants additional investigation.

5   Notes

1. **Tumor models**: Female Sprague–Dawley rats (5 weeks old), male ddY mice (6 weeks old), female BALB/c mice (6 weeks old), and male C57BL/6 J mice (6 weeks old) were purchased from SLC (Shizuoka, Japan). Rats were housed three per cage,

and mice were housed four or five per cage. For all animals, conditions were maintained at 22 ± 1 °C and 55 ± 5 % relative humidity with a 12-h light/dark cycle. All experiments were carried out according to the Laboratory Protocol for Animal Handling of Sojo University.

2. **Tumors:** Mouse S-180 sarcoma cells, from ascites maintained by weekly passage, were implanted subcutaneously (s.c.) in the dorsal skin of ddY mice, to obtain the S-180 tumor model. Mouse fibrosarcoma Meth-A cells (2×10^6) were maintained by intraperitoneal (i.p.) passage and then implanted s.c. in BALB/c mice. Colon adenocarcinoma C38 cells (2×10^6), purchased from the Riken Cell Bank (Tsukuba, Japan), were implanted s.c. in C57BL/6 mice. In addition, rat breast cancer was induced by oral administration of 10 mg of DMBA (a carcinogen) in 1 mL of corn oil. Bacterial distribution studies were started when the tumor diameters were 5–10 mm.

3. **Preparation of NG:** NG ointment contained 20 mg/g Vaseline® and was used after 10- or 100-fold dilution with Vaseline®.

4. **Evans blue:** When injected into circulation, it binds to albumin to form a complex of about 69 kDa and is thus considered a putative macromolecular drug.

5. **PEG-conjugated zinc protoporphyrin IX (ZnPP) (PZP):** The synthesis, purification, and characterization of PZP were previously described [51]. PZP consists of two chains of PEG, each about 2,500 Da, conjugated to ZnPP to form micelles of about 180 nm in diameter, and a mean molecular mass of about 110 kDa determined by size-exclusion chromatography. Radiolabeled PZP was obtained by utilizing ^{65}Zn during the zinc insertion step of PZP synthesis [52].

6. *Lactobacillus* **bacteria:** *L. casei* strain Shirota was cultured in MRS (de Man, Rogosa, Sharpe) medium. Lactulose (4-*O*-β-D-galactopyranosyl-D-fructofuranose), was used during in vivo experiments with *L. casei* [6].

Acknowledgment

This work was supported in part by a Grant-in-Aid from the Ministry of Education, Science, Culture, Sports and Technology of Japan (No. 08011717), a Cancer Speciality grant from the Ministry of Health, Welfare and Labour (H23-Third Term Comprehensive Control Research, General-001), and research funds of the Faculty of Pharmaceutical Sciences at Sojo University.

References

1. Matsumura Y, Maeda H (1986) A new concept for macromolecular therapeutics in cancer chemotherapy: mechanism of tumoritropic accumulation of proteins and the antitumor agent smancs. Cancer Res 46:6387–6392
2. Lammers T (2012) Drug delivery research in Europe. J Control Release 161:151
3. Seki T, Fang J, Maeda H (2009) Tumor targeted macromolecular drug delivery based on the enhanced permeability and retention effect in solid tumor. In: Lu Y, Mahato RI (eds) Pharmaceutical perspectives of cancer therapeutics. AAPS-Springer, New York, pp 93–102
4. Maeda H, Sawa T, Konno T (2001) Mechanism of tumor-targeted delivery of macromolecular drugs, including the EPR effect in solid tumor and clinical overview of the prototype polymeric drug SMANCS. J Control Release 74:47–61
5. Fang J, Nakamura H, Maeda H (2011) The EPR effect: unique features of tumor blood vessels for drug delivery, factors involved, and limitations and augmentation of the effect. Adv Drug Deliv Rev 63:136–151
6. Kimura NT, Taniguchi S, Aoki K et al (1980) Selective localization and growth of Bifidobacterium bifidum in mouse tumors following intravenous administration. Cancer Res 40:2061–2068
7. Hoffman RM (2009) Tumor-targeting amino acid auxotrophic Salmonella typhimurium. Amino Acids 37:509–521
8. Coley WB (1906) Late results of the treatment of inoperable sarcoma by the mixed toxins of erysipelas and Bacillus prodigiosus. Am J Med Sci 131:375–430
9. Malmgren RA, Flanigan CC (1955) Localization of the vegetative form of Clostridium tetani in mouse tumors following intravenous spore administration. Cancer Res 15:473–478
10. Möse JR, Möse G (1964) Oncolysis by clostridia. I. Activity of Clostridium butyricum (M-55) and other nonpathogenic clostridia against the Ehrlich carcinoma. Cancer Res 24:212–216
11. Kohwi Y, Imai K, Tamura Z et al (1978) Antitumor effect of Bifidobacterium infantis in mice. Gan 69:613–618
12. Brown JM, Giaccia AJ (1998) The unique physiology of solid tumors: opportunities (and problems) for cancer therapy. Cancer Res 58:1408–1416
13. Fox ME, Lemmon MJ, Mauchline ML et al (1996) Anaerobic bacteria as a delivery system for cancer gene therapy: in vitro activation of 5-fluorocytosine by genetically engineered clostridia. Gene Ther 3:173–178
14. Sznol M, Lin SL, Bermudes D et al (2000) Use of preferentially replicating bacteria for the treatment of cancer. J Clin Invest 105:1027–1030
15. Low KB, Ittensohn M, Le T et al (1999) Lipid A mutant Salmonella with suppressed virulence and TNFα induction retain tumor-targeting in vivo. Nat Biotechnol 17:37–41
16. Clairmont C, Lee KC, Pike J et al (2000) Biodistribution and genetic stability of the novel antitumor agent VNP20009, a genetically modified strain of Salmonella typhimurium. J Infect Dis 181:1996–2002
17. Yazawa K, Fujimori M, Amano J et al (2000) Bifidobacterium longum as a delivery system for cancer gene therapy: selective localization and growth in hypoxic tumors. Cancer Gene Ther 7:269–274
18. Zhao M, Yang M, Li XM et al (2005) Tumor-targeting bacterial therapy with amino acid auxotrophs of GFP-expressing Salmonella typhimurium. Proc Natl Acad Sci U S A 102:755–760
19. Xiang S, Fruehauf J, Li CJ (2006) Short hairpin RNA–expressing bacteria elicit RNA interference in mammals. Nat Biotechnol 24:697–702
20. Sasaki T, Fujimori M, Hamaji Y et al (2006) Genetically engineered Bifidobacterium longum for tumor-targeting enzyme-prodrug therapy of autochthonous mammary tumors in rats. Cancer Sci 97:649–657
21. Nanno M, Kato I, Kobayashi T et al (2011) Biological effects of probiotics: what impact does Lactobacillus casei Shirota have on us? Int J Immunopathol Pharmacol 24:45S–50S
22. Matsuzaki T (1998) Immunomodulation by treatment with Lactobacillus casei strain Shirota. Int J Food Microbiol 41:133–140
23. Suzuki F, Okabe H, Todaka T et al (1988) Heat-killed Lactobacillus casei, LC-9018, as an interferon inducer. Nihon Saikingaku Zasshi 43:821–827
24. Maeda H, Noguchi Y, Sato K et al (1994) Enhanced vascular permeability in solid tumor is mediated by nitric oxide and inhibited by both new nitric oxide scavenger and nitric oxide synthase inhibitor. Jpn J Cancer Res 85:331–334
25. Wu J, Akaike T, Maeda H (1998) Modulation of enhanced vascular permeability in tumors by a bradykinin antagonist, a cyclooxygenase inhibitor, and nitric oxide scavenger. Cancer Res 58:159–165
26. Maeda H, Nakamura H, Fang J (2013) The EPR effect for macromolecular drug delivery to solid tumors: improvement of tumor uptake,

lowering of systemic toxicity, and distinct tumor imaging in vivo. Adv Drug Deliv Rev 65:71–79

27. Fukuto JM, Cho JY, Switzer CH (2000) The chemical properties of nitric oxide and related nitrogen oxides. In: Ignarro LJ (ed) Nitric oxide: biology and pathobiology. Academic, San Diego, CA, pp 23–39

28. Feelisch M, Noack EA (1987) Correlation between nitric oxide formation during degradation of organic nitrates and activation of guanylate cyclase. Eur J Pharmacol 139:19–30

29. Chen Z, Stamler JS (2006) Bioactivation of nitroglycerin by the mitochondrial aldehyde dehydrogenase. Trends Cardiovasc Med 16:259–265

30. Seki T, Fang J, Maeda H (2009) Enhanced delivery of macromolecular antitumor drugs to tumors by nitroglycerin application. Cancer Sci 100:2426–2430

31. Maeda H (2010) Nitroglycerin enhances vascular blood flow and drug delivery in hypoxic tumor tissues: analogy between angina pectoris and solid tumors and enhancement of the EPR effect. J Control Release 142:296–298

32. Torchilin V (2011) Tumor delivery of macromolecular drugs based on the EPR effect. Adv Drug Deliv Rev 63:131–135

33. Vicent MJ, Ringsdorf H, Duncan R (2009) Polymer therapeutics: clinical applications and challenges for development. Adv Drug Deliv Rev 61:1117–1120

34. Matsumura Y, Kataoka K (2009) Preclinical and clinical studies of anticancer agent-incorporating polymer micelles. Cancer Sci 100:572–579

35. Noguchi Y, Wu J, Duncan R et al (1998) Early phase tumor accumulation of macromolecules: a great difference in clearance rate between tumor and normal tissues. Jpn J Cancer Res 89:307–314

36. Kato I, Kobayashi S, Yokokura T et al (1981) Antitumor activity of *Lactobacillus casei* in mice. Gan 72:517–523

37. Kato I, Yokokura T, Mutai M (1985) Induction of tumoricidal peritoneal exudate cells by administration of *Lactobacillus casei*. Int J Immunopharmacol 7:103–109

38. Kato I, Yokokura T, Mutai M (1983) Macrophage activation by *Lactobacillus casei* in mice. Microbiol Immunol 27:611–618

39. Kato I, Yokokura T, Mutai M (1984) Augmentation of mouse natural killer cell activity by *Lactobacillus casei* and its surface antigens. Microbiol Immunol 28:209–217

40. Ignarro LJ (2000) Nitric oxide: biology and pathobiology. Academic, San Diego, CA

41. Jordan BF, Misson PD, Demeure R et al (2000) Changes in tumor oxygenation/perfusion induced by the NO donor, isosorbide dinitrate, in comparison with carbogen: monitoring by EPR and MRI. Int J Radiat Oncol Biol Phys 48:565–570

42. Mitchell JB, Wink DA, DeGraff W et al (1993) Hypoxic mammalian cell radiosensitization by nitric oxide. Cancer Res 53:5845–5848

43. Yasuda H, Nakayama K, Watanabe M et al (2006) Nitroglycerin treatment may enhance chemosensitivity to docetaxel and carboplatin in patients with lung adenocarcinoma. Clin Cancer Res 12:6748–6757

44. Nagamitsu A, Greish K, Maeda H (2009) Elevating blood pressure as a strategy to increase tumor-targeted delivery of macromolecular drug SMANCS: cases of advanced solid tumors. Jpn J Clin Oncol 39:756–766

45. Tanaka S, Akaike T, Wu J et al (2003) Modulation of tumor-selective vascular blood flow and extravasation by the stable prostaglandin 12 analogue beraprost sodium. J Drug Target 11(1):45–52

46. Fang J, Qin H, Nakamura H et al (2012) Carbon monoxide, generated by heme oxygenase-1, mediates the enhanced permeability and retention effect in solid tumors. Cancer Sci 103:535–541

47. Aso Y, Akaza H, Kotake T et al (1995) Preventive effect of a *Lactobacillus casei* preparation on the recurrence of superficial bladder cancer in a double-blind trial. The BLP Study Group. Eur Urol 27:104–109

48. Ohashi Y, Nakai S, Tsukamoto T et al (2002) Habitual intake of lactic acid bacteria and risk reduction of bladder cancer. Urol Int 68:273–280

49. Sylvester RJ, van der Meijden AP, Lamm DL (2002) Intravesical bacillus Calmette-Guerin reduces the risk of progression in patients with superficial bladder cancer: a meta-analysis of the published results of randomized clinical trials. J Urol 168:1964–1970

50. Fang J, Liao L, Yin H, Nakamura H, Shin T, Maeda H (2014) Enhanced bacterial tumor delivery by modulating the EPR effect and therapeutic potential of Lactobacillus casei. J Pharm Sci 103:3235–3243

51. Sahoo SK, Sawa T, Fang J et al (2002) Pegylated zinc protoporphyrin: a water-soluble heme oxygenase inhibitor with tumor-targeting capacity. Bioconjug Chem 13:1031–1038

52. Fang J, Sawa T, Akaike T et al (2003) In vivo antitumor activity of pegylated zinc protoporphyrin: targeted inhibition of heme oxygenase in solid tumor. Cancer Res 63:3567–3574

Chapter 3

Oral Delivery of Tumor-Targeting *Salmonella* to Treat Cancer in Mice

Dongping Wei and Lijun Jia

Abstract

Tumor-targeting bacteria have been developed as novel anticancer agents recently. To achieve their therapeutic effects, bacteria have conventionally been injected intravenously or intraperitoneally into animals or humans. Here, we describe the oral delivery of tumor-targeting *Salmonella* for cancer therapy in a mouse tumor model. We detail the experimental procedures for establishing a mouse tumor model, preparing bacterial culture, mouse gavage, and detection of the tumor-targeting capability of bacteria administered orally. We also discuss technical notes and provide practical advice that will help the users of this oral delivery model.

Key words Oral delivery, Tumor-targeting bacteria, *Salmonella*, Solid tumor, Cancer therapy

1 Introduction

Tumor-targeting bacteria have been emerging as therapeutic agents against solid tumors. To achieve their therapeutic effects, bacteria have conventionally been injected intra-venously or intra-peritoneally into animals or humans [1–14]. However, the systemic administration of bacteria is inconvenient and also carries the risk of toxicity. To overcome these disadvantages, we have previously established an alternative infection model, in which tumor-targeting *Salmonella* can be orally administered to mice bearing subcutaneous tumors [15–17]. We found that orally-delivered *Salmonella* exhibited high tumor-targeting potential and did not compromise its therapeutic efficacy [15–17]. Importantly, oral administration of the tumor-targeting *Salmonella* demonstrated minimal toxicity in mice compared to systemic infection, indicating a high safety profile of the oral delivery route [15–17]. To facilitate the use of this system as a preclinical model for bacteria-based cancer therapies, we detail here the experimental protocol for oral delivery of tumor-targeting *Salmonella* to treat cancer using a mouse tumor model. The critical steps of the procedure

Robert M. Hoffman (ed.), *Bacterial Therapy of Cancer: Methods and Protocols*, Methods in Molecular Biology, vol. 1409, DOI 10.1007/978-1-4939-3515-4_3, © Springer Science+Business Media New York 2016

described include (1) establishment of a mouse tumor model; (2) bacterial enumeration; (3) oral gavage with bacteria in mice; and (4) bacteria isolation and titration post treatment. We also discuss technical notes and provide practical advice that will help the users of this oral delivery model. When the protocol is followed correctly, the preferential accumulation of *Salmonella* within tumors should be observed, which is basically responsible for the significant anti-cancer activity of the bacteria in tumor-bearing mice.

2   Materials

All solutions used in this study are prepared by using ultra-pure water (prepared by purifying de-ionized water to attain a sensitivity of 18 MΩ cm at 25 °C) and analytical grade reagents.

1 mL syringe with 22.5 G needle.

Oral gavage needle (18 G) with a bulb tip.

Six micro-cuvettes.

Spectrophotometer.

Bacterial spreader.

Bacterial strain: Lipid A-modified (*msbB−*), auxotrophic (*purI−*) *Salmonella typhimurium* VNP20009 (VNP20009) is obtained from the American Type Culture Collection (ATCC).

Modified-LB broth for VNP20009 culture: 10 g tryptone, 5 g yeast extract, 2 mL 1 N $CaCl_2$, and 2 mL 1 N $MgSO_4$ per liter, adjusted to pH 7 using 1 N NaOH (*see* **Note 1**).

B16F10 melanoma cells are obtained from the ATCC, and cultured as a monolayer in Dulbecco's Modified Eagle's Medium (DMEM) supplemented with 10 % fetal bovine serum (FBS). The cells are verified as being free of mycoplasma contamination (*see* **Note 2**). Cell cultures are maintained in an atmosphere of 5 % CO_2/95 % air at 37 °C.

C57BL/6J mice used for the study: 6- to 8-week-old female C57BL/6J (18–20 g). Mice are housed in a biosafety-level-2 (BSL-2) containment facility (*see* **Note 3**).

3   Methods

3.1   Establishment of a Mouse Tumor Model

1. Grow B16F10 cells to 80–90 % confluence.

2. Wash with PBS (pH 7.4), trypsinize, and suspend with DMEM containing 10 % FBS.

3. Spin down the cell pellets, suspend and make a concentration of 5×10^6 cells/mL using PBS (pH 7.4).

4. Inject subcutaneously (s.c.) 5×10^5 B16F10 cells (in 0.1 mL PBS) per mouse into the right flank using a 1 mL syringe with a 22.5 G needle (*see* **Note 4**).

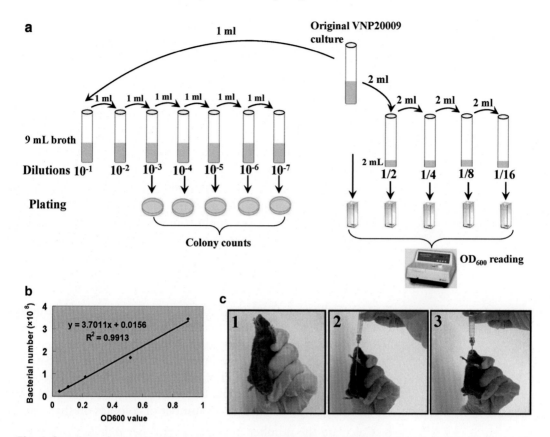

Fig. 1 Overview of procedure for mouse oral gavage treatment with tumor-targeting *Salmonella*. (**a**) The VNP20009 culture was diluted by tenfold and twofold serial dilutions. While the tenfold dilution series were plated onto agar plates for colony counts, the two-fold dilution series were used for spectrophotometric analysis. (**b**) Correlation of optical density with viable plate count. (**c**) Oral gavage. The mouse was properly restrained with the left hand (*1*), and the length of the gavage needle against the animal's body was measured (*2*). The bacterial inoculum was orally administered to the mouse upon verification of proper placement of the gavage needle (*3*)

5. Monitor the tumor every other day. When the average tumor volume reaches approximately 150 mm³, randomize the mice for oral gavage as described in the next section.

3.2 Bacteria Enumeration

The bacterial number is determined by performing a viable plate count and measuring the optical density of the bacterial suspension (Fig. 1).

3.2.1 Viable Plate Count

1. Prepare sufficient modified-LB broth and agar plates required for the study and store at 4 °C until used.

2. Culture VNP20009 on the modified-LB agar plate and incubate at 37 °C overnight.

3. Pick a clone of VNP20009 from the modified-LB agar plate and place into 3 mL modified-LB broth in a 12 mL tube, and shake at 225 rpm, 37 °C overnight (~16 h).

4. Dilute the overnight VNP20009 culture into modified LB at a ratio of 1:100, grow with shaking at 37 °C, until the optical density at wavelength 600 nm (OD_{600}) reaches 0.8–1.0 and chill on ice.

5. Set up seven dilution tubes, each containing 9 mL sterile modified LB.

6. Aseptically transfer 1 mL VNP20009 culture into the first tube to make a 10^{-1} dilution (keep the original tube of VNP20009 culture on ice for spectrophotometric analysis) by using a pipette with a sterile tip. Discard the pipette tip. Mix thoroughly and transfer 1 mL of bacterial suspension to the next dilution tube (10^{-2} dilution) with a fresh pipette tip. Proceed in this way in order to obtain a 10^{-7} dilution (Fig. 1a).

7. Aseptically transfer 0.1 mL of the last five bacterial dilutions (from 10^{-3} to 10^{-7}) onto a corresponding agar plate in triplicate. Spread the liquid over the whole surface of the plate by using a spreader. Once dry, invert all the plates and incubate at 37 °C for 24 h. At the end of the incubation period, select the plates that appear to contain between 30 and 300 colonies (*see* **Note 5**) and count the exact number of colonies on that plate.

8. Calculate the number of bacteria (cfu) per milliliter of sample by dividing the number of colonies by the dilution factor multiplied by the amount of bacterial suspension plated on an agar plate.

3.2.2 Spectrophotometric Analysis

1. Place the original tube of VNP20009 and four tubes of 2 mL sterile modified LB in a test-tube rack.

2. Use four of these tubes (tubes 2–5) of broth to make twofold serial dilution of the bacterial culture to produce 1/2, 1/4, 1/8, and 1/16 dilutions (Fig. 1a).

3. Pipette 1 mL of the sterile modified LB into one of the micro-cuvettes and standardize the spectrophotometer as directed. Pipette 1 mL of the original VNP20009 culture into a second micro-cuvette and place in the machine and read the OD_{600} value. Repeat this with the 1/2, 1/4, 1/8, and 1/16 dilutions. Record the OD_{600} values along with the dilutions that they originated from (Table 1).

3.2.3 Correlate the OD_{600} Value with Viable Plate Count

1. Calculate the approximate numbers of bacteria in the 1/2, 1/4, 1/8, and 1/16 dilutions by halving the bacterial number shown in Table 1.

2. Plot these five coordinates on a graph using EXCEL software with a formula (Fig. 1b) that is used for converting OD_{600} values into bacterial counts (CFU/mL) (*see* **Note 6**).

Table 1
Bacteria enumeration

Dilution	OD_{600} (x axis)	Bacterial number (y axis)
Original	0.899	3.45×10^8
1/2	0.519	1.73×10^8
1/4	0.218	0.86×10^8
1/8	0.104	0.43×10^8
1/16	0.045	0.22×10^8

3.3 Bacterial Inoculum Preparation

1. Dilute the overnight VNP20009 culture into modified LB at a ratio of 1:100 and grow to an OD_{600} of 0.8–1.0 and chill on ice.

2. Estimate the concentration (CFU/mL) of the VNP20009 culture with the formula shown in Fig. 1b.

3. Transfer the desired volume of the VNP20009 culture to a falcon tube and centrifuge at $3500 \times g$ for 15 min.

4. Wash the bacterial pellet with PBS and resuspend in PBS such that the bacterial inoculum is 1×10^{10} CFU/mL.

3.4 Oral Gavage

All animal experiments were carried out according to a protocol approved by the Fudan University Committee for Use and Care of Animals.

1. Fast the mice for 4 h prior to oral gavage.

2. Manually restrain the animal by grasping the mouse skin over the shoulder firmly with the thumb and forefingers to immobilize the head and torso (Fig. 1c).

3. Gently stretch the head with the forefingers finger to make the esophagus extended, which creates a straight line through the neck and esophagus.

4. Keep the animal in an upright position and then measure the distance from the tip of the nose to the last rib on the left side by using the needle held next to the animal (Fig. 1c). This is the approximate distance to the stomach and the needle should not be advanced further than that distance to avoid perforating the stomach.

5. Direct the ball tip of the oral gavage needle along the roof of the mouth and toward the right side of the back of the pharynx (*see* **Note 7**), then gently pass into the esophagus and inject the 100 µl (*see* **Note 8**) bacterial inoculum (1×10^9 CFU).

6. Return the animal to the cage and monitor for 5–10 min, looking for any sign of labored breathing or distress (*see* **Note 9**).

7. Feed the mice with adequate food and drinking water after oral gavage of bacteria.

3.5 Bacteria Isolation and Titration

1. Aseptically remove and weigh tumors, livers, and spleens from tumor-bearing mice on days 7, 14, and 21 post treatment.

2. Homogenize tissue with ice-cold, sterile PBS (pH 7.4) at a ratio of 5:1 (PBS volume (mL): tissue weight (g)).

3. Centrifuge at $800 \times g$ for 10 min. Transfer the supernatant into a clean 12 mL tube.

4. Serially dilute the homogenates in the range of 10^{-1} to 10^{-8}.

5. Spread each dilution onto a modified-LB agar plate in triplicate and incubate at 37 °C for 24 h.

6. Count plates that have between 30 and 300 colonies.

7. Determine the titer of bacteria (CFU/g tissue) by counting colonies and dividing them by the weight of the tissue (Fig. 2a). Tumor-targeting by VNP20009 can be calculated as the ratio of the bacteria titer between the tumor and liver.

3.6 Assessment of Antitumor Efficacy and Potential Toxicity of Orally Delivered Salmonella

1. Monitor tumor growth to evaluate the inhibitory efficacy of orally-administered VNP20009 in tumor-bearing mice. Measure tumors individually with a caliper. Determine tumor volumes by the formula: tumor volume = length × width^2 × 0.52 (Fig. 2b).

2. Orally administer 1×10^9 cfu VNP20009 to tumor-free mice and determine body weight change at different time points, as indicated (Fig. 2c).

4 Notes

1. Distinct bacterial species or bacterial strains have their own growth requirements. In the case of *Salmonella typhimurium* VNP20009 (*msbB⁻purI⁻*), it should be grown either in LB broth containing no salt or in modified LB as shown in Subheading 3 in order to avoid spontaneous variants of the *msbB⁻* mutants.

2. Sometimes tumors will spontaneously regress due to cell-line contamination with mycoplasma. Therefore, it is necessary to make sure that the cell line used for a xenograft study is free of mycoplasma contamination.

3. If mice are obtained from an external supplier, it is advised to feed the mice for 1 week, following transport to the facility, with autoclaved food and water in order to stabilize the gut microbiota.

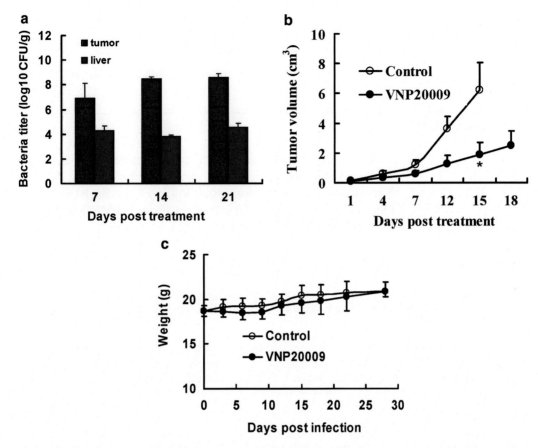

Fig. 2 Antitumor efficacy and safety of orally-administered tumor-targeting *Salmonella*. (**a**) Orally-delivered *Salmonella* selectively accumulated in tumors. C57BL/6 mice bearing B16F10 melanoma were orally administrated with VNP20009 (10^9 CFU/mouse). Bacterial titers in tumors and livers were determined at 7, 14, 21 days post treatment ($n = 3–4$). (**b**) Orally administrated *Salmonella* significantly inhibited tumor growth in mice. *$P < 0.001$. (**c**) Orally-administered *Salmonella* did not cause significant body-weight loss compared to the control mice during a 1-month treatment period ($P > 0.05$)

4. Because the small-bore needle may produce shear stress on the cells, causing them to rupture, it is advised that a narrow gauge needle should not be used for cancer cell inoculation.

5. Fewer than 30 colonies are not statistically valid, while more than 300 colonies on a plate are likely to produce colonies too close to each other to be distinguished as distinct colony-forming units.

6. This formula has been made based on our experimental setting and will not be valid if the parameters (e.g., culture media, bacteria, and spectrophotometer) used to obtain the formula changes.

7. If any resistance is encountered to gavage, you may be attempting to enter the trachea. You need to stop and gently remove the needle to avoid injecting fluid into the lungs.

8. In general, the maximum volume administered to a mouse by oral gavage should not exceed 1 % of the body weight because of the anatomical limitation of gastric distension.

9. If fluid is injected in the lungs, the mice should be euthanized.

Acknowledgement

We thank Lihui Li and Xiaoxin Zhang for their technical assistance. This study was supported by grants from the Chinese National Natural Science Foundation (30500637 to Lijun Jia; 81472793 to Dongping Wei) and Key Project of the Shanghai Municipal Health Bureau (2010012 to Lijun Jia).

References

1. Yazawa K, Fujimor IM, Amano J, Kano Y, Taniguchi S (2000) Bifidobacterium longum as a delivery system for cancer gene therapy: selective localization and growth in hypoxic tumors. Cancer Gene Ther 7:269–274

2. Lee CH, Wu CL, Shiau AL (2004) Endostatin gene therapy delivered by Salmonella choleraesuis in murine tumor models. J Gene Med 6:1382–1393

3. Zheng LM, Luo X, Feng M et al (2000) Tumor amplified protein expression therapy: Salmonella as a tumor-selective protein delivery vector. Oncol Res 12:127–135

4. King I, Bermudes D, Lin S et al (2002) Tumor-targeted Salmonella expressing cytosine deaminase as an anticancer agent. Hum Gene Ther 13:1225–1233

5. Dang LH, Bettegowda C, Huso DL, Kinzler KW, Vogelstein B (2001) Combination bacteriolytic therapy for the treatment of experimental tumors. Proc Natl Acad Sci USA 98:15155–15160

6. Dang LH, Bettegowda C, Agrawal N et al (2004) Targeting vascular and avascular compartments of tumors with C. novyi-NT and anti-microtubule agents. Cancer Biol Ther 3:326–337

7. Lee CH, Wu CL, Tai YS, Shiau AL (2005) Systemic administration of attenuated Salmonella choleraesuis in combination with cisplatin for cancer therapy. Mol Ther 11:707–716

8. Chen J, Wei D, Zhuang H, Qiao Y, Tang B, Zhang X, Wei J, Fang S, Chen G, Du P, Huang X, Jiang W, Hu Q, Hua ZC (2011) Proteomic screening of anaerobically regulated promoters from Salmonella and its antitumor applications. Mol Cell Proteomics 10:M111.009399

9. Bettegowda C, Dang LH, Abrams R et al (2003) Overcoming the hypoxic barrier to radiation therapy with anaerobic bacteria. Proc Natl Acad Sci USA 100:15083–15088

10. Jia LJ, Xu HM, Ma DY et al (2005) Enhanced therapeutic effect by combination of tumor-targeting Salmonella and endostatin in murine melanoma model. Cancer Biol Ther 4:840–845

11. Tjuvajev J, Blasberg R, Luo X, Zheng LM, King I, Bermudes D (2001) Salmonella-based tumor-targeted cancer therapy: tumor amplified protein expression therapy (TAPET) for diagnostic imaging. J Control Release 74:313–315

12. Yu YA, Shabahang S, Timiryasova TM et al (2004) Visualization of tumors and metastases in live animals with bacteria and vaccinia virus encoding light-emitting proteins. Nat Biotechnol 22:313–320

13. Hayashi K, Zhao M, Yamauchi K, Yamamoto N, Tsuchiya H, Tomita K, Kishimoto H, Bouvet M, Hoffman RM (2009) Systemic targeting of primary bone tumor and lung metastasis of high-grade osteosarcoma in nude mice with a tumor-selective strain of Salmonella typhimurium. Cell Cycle 8:870–875

14. Zhang Y, Zhang N, Zhao M, Hoffman RM (2015) Comparison of the selective targeting efficacy of Salmonella typhimurium A1-R and VNP20009 on the Lewis lung carcinoma in nude mice. Oncotarget 6:14625–14631

15. Jia LJ, Wei DP, Sun QM, Huang Y, Wu Q, Hua ZC (2007) Oral delivery of tumor-targeting Salmonella for cancer therapy in murine tumor models. Cancer Sci 98:1107–1112

16. Chen G, Wei DP, Jia LJ, Tang B, Shu L, Zhang K, Xu Y, Gao J, Huang XF, Jiang WH, Hu QG, Huang Y, Wu Q, Sun ZH, Zhang JF, Hua ZC (2009) Oral delivery of tumor-targeting Salmonella exhibits promising therapeutic efficacy and low toxicity. Cancer Sci 100:2437–2443

17. Zhang Y, Tome Y, Suetsugu A, Zhang L, Zhang N, Hoffman R, Zhao M (2012) Determination of the optimal route of administration of *Salmonella typhimurium* A1-R to target breast cancer in nude mice. Anticancer Res 32:2501–2508

Chapter 4

Microfluidic Device to Quantify the Behavior of Therapeutic Bacteria in Three-Dimensional Tumor Tissue

Emily L. Brackett, Charles A. Swofford, and Neil S. Forbes

Abstract

Microfluidic devices enable precise quantification of the interactions between anti-cancer bacteria and tumor tissue. Direct observation of bacterial movement and gene expression in tissue is difficult with either monolayers of cells or tumor-bearing mice. Quantification of these interactions is necessary to understand the inherent mechanisms of bacterial targeting and to develop modified organisms with enhanced therapeutic properties. Here we describe the procedures for designing, printing, and assembling microfluidic tumor-on-a-chip devices. We also describe the procedures for inserting three-dimensional tumor-cell masses, exposure to bacteria, and analyzing the resultant images.

Key words Microfluidic device, Tumor-on-a-chip, Tumor-targeting bacteria, PDMS, Cancer, Penetration, Motility, Accumulation, Lithography

1 Introduction

Microfluidic devices are invaluable for understanding the mechanisms that control bacterial interaction with tumors [1]. Therapeutic bacteria have many advantages over standard chemotherapeutic drugs because of their unique properties [2]. In vivo, bacteria preferentially accumulate in tumors over other organs [3] and actively penetrate through tumor tissue [4]. Bacteria have also been engineered to produce anti-cancer agents inside tumors [5]. However, poor understanding of these mechanisms has slowed development of these therapies. It is not possible to study tumor accumulation and penetration in monolayers of cancer cells, because they do not contain microenvironment gradients or barriers to mass transfer [6]. Experiments with mice are costly, time consuming, and cannot be easily used to measure dynamic behavior [4]. Microfluidic devices are essential tools for quantifying bacteria behavior, because they are cheap, fast, and can be imaged in real time. Microfluidic devices are also essential components in the development of new therapeutic strategies, because they can

Robert M. Hoffman (ed.), *Bacterial Therapy of Cancer: Methods and Protocols*, Methods in Molecular Biology, vol. 1409,
DOI 10.1007/978-1-4939-3515-4_4, © Springer Science+Business Media New York 2016

rapidly evaluate genetic modifications that have been designed to improve bacterial performance.

Here we describe a procedure to create a microfluidic device that contains a tissue chamber with a flow channel on one side (Fig. 1). This geometry exposes the contained cells to flowing medium, mimicking the interaction between cells and blood vessels [3]. The device is formed by imprinting a design in polydimethylsiloxane (PDMS), and adhering it to glass [7, 8]. Cancer cells are inserted as spheroids and retained by a filter at the rear of the chamber [7]. The geometry of the device ensures that the cell mass is optically accessible through a glass slide (Fig. 2). Because the design is vertically uniform (away from the glass), mass transfer creates linear microenvironment gradients that are identical in all

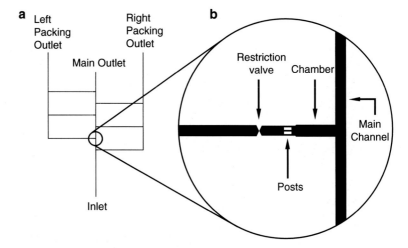

Fig. 1 Schematic of microfluidic chamber and channels. (**a**) Basic device containing a main channel with six alternating chambers connecting a main outlet and two packing outlets. (**b**) Enlarged view highlighting the main channel, one chamber, posts, and restriction valve

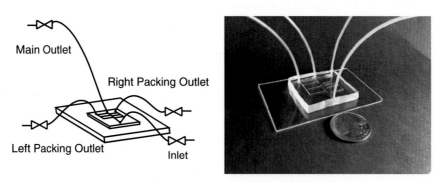

Fig. 2 Schematic of device assembly and tubing. The device is comprised of a PDMS layer adhered to a glass slide with tubing attached to the main outlet, the packing outlets, and the inlet. Actual size, shown relative to a quarter

z-planes. This uniformity enables analysis by standard epifluorescence microscopy [7].

Using this device, we have shown that bacterial motility is necessary for deep penetration into tumor tissue and that motile species are more effective at colonization [1]. Using a similar device, we have shown that chemotaxis and growth are necessary mechanisms for *Salmonella* accumulation in tumors [9, 10]. Chemoreceptors attract bacteria to specific microenvironments created by dying cancer cells [10]. The ability to observe a live population in real time, permits modeling of the bacterial behavior and precise quantification of chemotaxis and growth [9]. Other groups have used similar devices to show that *Salmonella* have a preference for liver cancer cells compared to normal cells [11], and expression of *invasin* increases proliferation of *E. coli* in 3D tumor tissue [12].

A microfluidic device could be used to answer many unanswered questions about how bacteria interact with tumors. Devices could be used to study (1) penetration into tissue, (2) invasion into cancer cells, (3) production of drug molecules, and (4) control of gene expression. In addition, the response of cancer cells to invasion and bacterially-produced molecules could be quantified in real time. A microfluidic device would be an essential component in the design of more effective bacteria by enabling visualization of engineered improvements in penetration, invasion, and drug production.

The procedure below outlines the steps necessary to design, fabricate and run a microfluidic device. The description is focused on a specific design with a single inlet, two outlets, and a tissue-containing chamber. We have found this design to be simple to implement and stable for multiple days [7]. However, this soft-lithography technique is highly flexible and could be tuned for multiple applications by designing different architectures. The procedure is made up of four basic phases: (1) design and construction of the microfluidic device (Subheadings 3.1–3.5); (2) growth and insertion of cancer cells (Subheadings 3.6 and 3.7); (3) treatment with bacteria (Subheading 3.8); and (4) image acquisition and analysis (Subheading 3.9).

2 Materials

2.1 Mold and Device

1. 4 in. diameter, 525 μm thick silicon wafers (*University Wafer*, South Boston, MA, USA).

2. SU-8 2050 permanent epoxy-negative photoresist and developer (*Microchem*, Newton, MA, USA).

3. 150×5 mm polystyrene petri dishes covered in aluminum foil, as light-block covers.

4. 100 % silicone rubber, 732 multipurpose sealant (*Dow Corning*, Midland, MI, USA).

5. Sylgard 184 silicone elastomer kit: silicone elastomer base and curing agent (*Dow Corning*).

6. 1.5 mm biopsy punch drill bit.

7. Microbore PTFE 0.032 in. ID, 0.056 in. OD tubing.

8. Super Flangeless Fittings system, Tefzel, 1/16″ OD (*Upchurch Scientific*, Oak Harbor, WA, USA).

9. 0.040 thru shut-off valve (*Upchurch Scientific*, Oak Harbor, WA, USA).

2.2 Mammalian-Cell and Bacterial Culture

1. Low-glucose medium: low-glucose Dulbecco's Modified Eagle Medium (DMEM) with 10 % fetal bovine serum (FBS), pH adjusted to 7.4, sterile filtered, and stored at 4 °C.

2. HEPES-buffered medium: low-glucose DMEM with 10 % FBS and 6 g/L HEPES buffer.

3. PMMA/ethanol solution: In a cell-culture hood, add 20 g/L poly(methyl methacrylate) to pure ethanol. Store at 37 °C and 5 % carbon dioxide.

4. Phosphate-buffered saline (PBS) without calcium or magnesium.

5. 0.05 % trypsin–EDTA 1× phenol red.

6. LB medium: To 950 mL Nanopure water, add 10 g tryptone, 5 g yeast extract, and 10 g sodium chloride. Use sodium hydroxide to adjust the pH to 7.0. Sterilize by autoclaving at 15 psi for 20 min. Store at room temperature.

3 Methods

When working with silicon wafers, use tweezers and avoid touching any area on the wafer. When the device is not in use for longer than an hour, cover it with plastic wrap.

3.1 Device Design

1. Draw design using a vector drawing program (*see* **Note 1**).

2. In the design, connect chambers to flow inlets and outlets at the front of the chamber and packing outlets on the rear of chamber. Chambers are 1000×300 µm, channels are 250 µm, posts are 195×65 µm, and restriction valves are a triangle and an inverted triangle spanning a 125×250 µm area (*see* Fig. 1 and **Note 2**).

3. Print devices on high quality imagesetting film with 100 µm polyester base and 5080 dpi resolution (*see* **Note 3**).

3.2 Mold Fabrication

1. Using tweezers, wash each silicon wafer twice with toluene, isopropanol, and water. Spray solvents over entire surface and dry completely between solvents, using air.

2. Center wafer on spin coater and apply vacuum. Pour approximately 4 mL SU-8 2050 onto the center of wafer. Spin at 500 rpm for 10 s with an acceleration of 100 rpm/s (**step 1**) then at 1250 rpm for 30 s with an acceleration of 300 rpm/s (**step 2**). These steps will achieve a thickness of 150 μm with SU-8 2050. Minimize light exposure during spin coating to avoid decomposition of SU-8.

3. Release vacuum and remove wafer using tweezers. Place wafer on a 65 °C slide heater, under a light-blocking plastic lid, and on top of a laboratory wipe for 5 min.

4. Remove wafer and allow to cool for 5 min. During this cooling step, increase heater setting to 95 °C. Place wafer back onto the heater for 30 min. Remove wafer again and allow to cool completely (*see* **Note 4**).

5. In a minimally-lit area, securely attach design transparency on top of wafer using paper clips. Avoid bubbles, dust, tweezers marks, and other imperfections on the wafer sections. Cover any remaining exposed wafer surface with tin foil to ensure only desired features are exposed. An exposure of 260 mJ/cm² is recommended for ideal cross-linking. For example, with a UV reading of 13.18 MW/cm², a single exposure of 20 s is used (*see* **Note 5**).

6. Again, heat wafer to 65 °C for 5 min while covered (*see* **Step 4**), cool for 5 min, and heat to 95 °C for 12 min. Remove wafer and allow it to cool completely.

7. Using tweezers, place wafer on top of a magnetic stir bar in a high-walled glass dish. Add enough SU-8 2050 developer to just cover wafer. Turn magnetic stirrer to lowest setting for approximately 25 min. To verify that SU-8 2050 is completely developed, remove wafer using tweezers and spray with isopropanol. If a milky deposit forms, dry wafer with air and return to the developer. Once fully developed, clean wafer with isopropanol and dry with air.

8. Glue wafer to a plastic petri dish. Apply a circle of 100 % silicone sealant approximately 1 cm from the features. Allow 24 h for sealant to set before use.

3.3 Device Fabrication

1. Mix 10.8 g PDMS and 1.2 g silicone curing agent in a 50 mL centrifuge tube. Vortex on high for 1 min. Pour mixture into mold, allowing as little as possible to spill over sealant edges (*see* **Note 6**).

2. To de-gas PDMS solution, cycle between applying and releasing vacuum suction within a vacuum chamber. When releasing vacuum, do so before bubbles spill over sealant edges. Continue until no bubbles are present on the wafer surface or over any features. Some bubbles may remain near sealant edges.

3. Place mold with lid on a slide heater at 65 °C for at least 5 h, preferably overnight.

4. Once cured, cut device away from mold using a scalpel and spatula, leaving approximately 0.5 cm edges from any desired features (*see* Fig. 2).

5. Wrap the device in plastic. Mark ends of each channel on plastic wrap with a dot. Punch these holes manually using a 1.5 mm biopsy punch (*see* **Note 7**).

6. Carefully remove debris using tweezers and a small needle. Clean with ethanol and air.

3.4 Plasma Treatment

1. Wash both device and a glass slide with acetone, isopropanol, and methanol in that order. Air-dry completely between solvents.

2. Place device and glass slide inside an oxygen plasma cleaner with bonding surfaces face up.

3. Cycle between vacuum and oxygen to purge air from the chamber. Open vacuum valve and allow pressure to drop to 200 mTorr. Open oxygen valve and allow pressure to return to 1 atm. Close oxygen valve and allow pressure to drop to 1 Torr. Open oxygen valve and allow pressure to return to 1 atm. Close oxygen valve and allow pressure to drop to 200 mTorr. Carefully open oxygen valve and balance oxygen and vacuum to maintain pressure at 200 mTorr.

4. Power on plasma cleaner and set to high for 2 min. A pink/purple glow should appear (*see* **Note 8**).

5. Power off the plasma cleaner, and close oxygen and vacuum valves. Once the door is able to open, gently but quickly place the two treated sides together. If necessary, gently tap device to induce bonding.

6. Wrap device with a laboratory wipe and place on a slide heater, glass-slide down. Put a glass jar, with a few hundred milliliters of water, on top as a weight. Leave at 65 °C for an hour. Wrap in plastic for storage.

3.5 Device Assembly

1. Cut seven 18-in. pieces and one 24 in. piece of PTFE tubing. At one end of each piece, attach a ferrule fitting. Screw each fitted end into a 0.040 thru-hole valve such that three valves have both ends of 18 in. tubing and one valve has one 18 in. tubing and one 24 in. tubing (*see* **Note 9**).

2. Attach the device to the bottom of a well plate with super glue and place on a microscope. Ensure that glue does not seep under the device around the features.

3. Arrange valves around the microscope such that the valve with 24 in. tubing is at least 11 in. above the device. Valves with all

18 in. tubing need not be arranged in any particular order (*see* **Note 10**).

4. Insert tubing from valves with 18 in. tubing into inlet and packing outlets of the device. Insert the 24 in. tubing to the main outlet (*see* Fig. 2).

5. In a cell-culture hood, fill three 10 mL syringes attached to 20 G, 1½ in. needles with 5–7 mL 70 % ethanol, 10 % bleach, and HEPES-buffered medium. Remove air bubbles by tapping syringes (*see* **Note 11**).

6. Open inlet valve and all outlet valves. Insert the ethanol syringe into the inlet tubing and gently push the syringe to flush the system. Close outlet valves and inlet valve in that order.

7. Repeat **step 6** with bleach and DMEM, in that order. Identify air bubbles and remove as many as possible during the medium flush. Do not inject entire medium syringe into the system as this will introduce air bubbles. Do not remove medium syringe attached to inlet tubing (*see* **Note 12**).

3.6 Cultivating Hanging-Drop Spheroids

1. Prepare a single-cell suspension of LS174T colon carcinoma cells by trypsinization. After centrifuging cells, resuspend pellet in 2–4 mL DMEM by pipetting up and down. Pipette vigorously with a micropipette to break up all cell clumps (*see* **Note 13**).

2. Count cell density using a hemocytometer, and create a 2 mL solution with a density of 300 cells/μL in DMEM.

3. Pipette 1 mL sterile water into each well of a 48-well plate. This water is critical for maintaining humidity and preventing evaporation of the small hanging drops.

4. Pipette 20 μL drops of cell and medium solution onto the inside surface of a well-plate lid. Gently touch the tip of a micropipette to just off center of each circle marked on the well plate lid. Inject cell-suspension medium toward the center of the marked circle (*see* Fig. 3 and **Note 14**).

5. Carefully turn lid over and place on well plate such that no drops touch well edges.

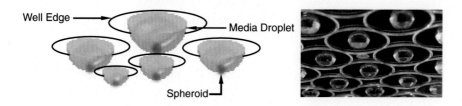

Fig. 3 Schematic and image of hanging drop spheroid formation. Spheroids are formed by suspending drops of medium from the lid of a well plate. Image shows LS174T tumor spheroids growing in media droplets, highlighting the well edge, media droplet, and spheroid

6. Incubate at 37 °C and 5 % carbon dioxide. Final spheroid size depends on length of culture time. Five days produces 500 μm diameter spheroids (*see* **Note 15**).

7. Prepare PMMA flasks in a cell-culture hood by adding approximately 1 mL of PMMA/ethanol solution to each T25 flask. Leave caps loose and allow ethanol to evaporate overnight in a cell-culture hood.

8. In a cell-culture hood, remove lid from hanging drop well plate and turn upside down. Using a 20 μL micropipette, select individual spheroids from drops. Add spheroids to a PMMA-coated T25 flask containing 5 mL DMEM (*see* **Note 16**).

9. Incubate for 5 days, until spheroids are 500 μm in diameter, which is optimal for insertion into the microfluidic device.

3.7 Spheroid Insertion

1. In a cell-culture hood, add 1 mL of spheroid-containing medium, from a PMMA-coated flask, into a 60 × 15 mm petri dish. Add 5 mL room-temperature HEPES-buffered medium to a second 60 × 15 mm petri dish.

2. Carefully select spheroids using a 20 μL micropipette and add them to the second dish. Select spheroids based on size, uniformity, symmetry and optical density (*see* **Note 17**).

3. Slowly draw spheroid-containing medium into a 10 mL syringe.

4. Attach a 20 G, 1½ in. needle to the syringe. With the needle facing up, allow spheroids to fall to the bottom of the syringe. Tap the syringe and gently push plunger to remove air bubbles.

5. With the needle facing down, allow spheroids to fall to the middle of the syringe. Lay the syringe on its side. Gently shake and roll syringe to move spheroids such that they do not contact each other.

6. Before injecting spheroids, ensure there are no air bubbles in the syringe. If so, repeat **steps 3** and **4** (*see* **Note 18**).

7. Remove the medium-containing syringe and attach a spheroid-containing syringe to tubing, while keeping the spheroid-containing syringe lying sideways.

8. Open inlet and packing outlets. Do not open main outlet (*see* Fig. 4a).

9. Run approximately 1–2 mL medium from the spheroid syringe through the device. Observe air bubbles and remove as many as possible. Do not inject spheroids into the system.

10. Turn the syringe and needle face down. Allow spheroids to fall into the needle. Gently push spheroids through the needle.

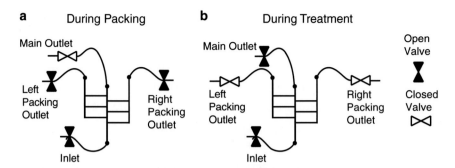

Fig. 4 Schematic of spheroid insertion. Valves are variably opened and closed during (**a**) spheroid insertion into chambers, and (**b**) delivery of treatment to the tumor tissue. (**a**) During insertion, the inlet and right and left packing outlet valves are open. (**b**) During treatment, the inlet and main outlet valves are open

Watch spheroids flow through tubing and into the inlet of the device (*see* **Note 19**).

11. Slowly push spheroids through the device using steady hand pressure. Injecting medium too quickly will cause spheroids to be shredded by posts at the rear of chambers and exit through packing outlets (*see* **Note 20**).

12. Once spheroids have been packed, stop pushing medium through the tubing but leave a thumb on the syringe to maintain pressure in the device. Close packing outlet valves followed by the inlet valve. Leave the spheroid syringe in the inlet tube.

13. Fill a 10 mL syringe, with an attached 20 G, 1½ in. needle, with 10 mL medium. Fit syringe into a syringe pump.

14. Start an automated image-acquisition process (*see* Subheading 3.9, **steps 1–3**).

15. Start the syringe pump with a flow rate of 3 μL/min. While watching spheroids through the microscope, slowly open the inlet valve, followed by the main outlet valve (*see* **Note 21**).

16. Inject medium into the device overnight to allow spheroids to grow into chambers.

3.8 Treatment with Bacteria

1. Grow bacteria in LB medium to mid-logarithmic phase ($0.2 < OD_{600} < 0.5$).

2. Centrifuge and resuspend bacteria in HEPES-buffered medium. Typical densities range from 10^5 to 10^7 CFU/mL.

3. Fill a 10 mL syringe attached to a 20 G, 1½ in. needle with bacteria solution.

4. Close main outlet valve followed by inlet valve. Stop the syringe pump.

5. Remove the medium syringe from the inlet valve and replace it with a bacteria syringe. Fit the bacteria syringe into the syringe pump.

6. Restart the syringe pump. While watching spheroids, slowly open inlet valve followed by main outlet valve.

7. Administer bacteria for 1 h (*see* **Note 22**).

8. Close main outlet valve followed by inlet valve. Stop the syringe pump program.

9. Remove bacteria syringe from inlet valve and replace it with a syringe containing only HEPES-buffered medium.

10. Fit medium syringe into syringe pump and restart it. While watching spheroids, slowly open inlet valve followed by main outlet valve.

3.9 Image Acquisition and Analysis and Time-lapse Images

1. Acquire images on an inverted microscope so that entire chamber, from rear to channel, is visible. If chamber is larger than a single image, tile multiple images together. Tiling requires alignment and calibration of an automated stage. Tiled images are created by acquiring an image, moving the stage one image width, and acquiring a second image (*see* **Note 23** and Fig. 5a).

2. Program the image acquisition sequence to acquire images of all six chambers in series for every time interval (*see* **Note 24**).

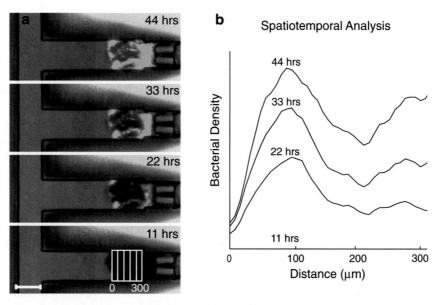

Fig. 5 *Salmonella* accumulated in tissue packed in the device. Results of bacterial treatment of one chamber. (**a**) Images of fluorescent bacteria (*green*) that have invaded into LS174T tumor tissue at four time points. Overlay on fourth image illustrates columns of pixels. The scale bar is 250 μm. (**b**) Profiles of bacterial density as a function of distance from the front of the tissue and as a function of time

3. After completion of the experiment, sort acquired images into individual stacks for each chamber. This creates a movie-like series of images.

4. For each chamber, rotate the images as a stack such that the rows of pixels line up with the edges of the chamber.

5. Identify the pixel columns that correspond to the front edge of the tissue and the rear of the chamber. Partition this area into columns of pixels (*see* Fig. 5a).

6. Average the fluorescence intensity of all pixels in each column individually from the front to the rear.

7. Convert pixel widths into absolute distances (i.e., micrometers).

8. This analysis on a stack of images creates an intensity profile as a function of distance for each image at each time point (*see* Fig. 5b).

9. Repeat for every chamber.

4   Notes

1. We use *Adobe* Illustrator to design our devices.

2. Our design has six chambers, three alternating on either side of one flow channel. The number of channels and the arrangement of the flow channels can easily be changed in the drawing process to match desired experimental protocols. Our device also has channels approximately 20 mm long, spaced 5 mm apart, with connecting outlet channels approximately 50 mm long to allow for stable features and leave room for the 1.5 mm biopsy-punch holes.

3. No stroke should be used when designing devices to make measurements as accurate as possible. Colors should be inverted before printing so that features appear white and space appears black. We send our designs to *PageWorks* (Cambridge, MA).

4. If heating the slide heater to 95 °C is not achievable during the 5 min cooling step, move on to the 30 min heating step regardless of the temperature of the heater. Do not allow the heater to go above 95 °C.

5. An energy meter can be used to gauge the lamp strength and appropriate exposure times may be selected based upon the energy output. Using one wafer and only a small section of the desired features to test multiple exposure times can effectively determine an ideal time. Under or over exposure can cause malformed device features.

6. The recommended weight ratio for a microfluidic device made from PDMS and a silicone curing agent is 10:1. However, a 9:1 ratio ensures the device will be stiff enough to hold the tubing during experiments. Any amount of the PDMS and curing agent mixture (i.e., above or below a total of 12 g) can be used, as long as the appropriate ratio is maintained for the desired stiffness.

7. Holes can be punched in a device by hand using the 1.5 mm biopsy drill bit. They can also be done with a drill press that is powered off. When using a drill, hold the device down firmly as you release the drill.

8. Settings should be adjusted for individual oxygen plasma cleaners. Times varying from 2 to 8 min have shown successful results, as well as pressures ranging from 200 to 150 mTorr.

9. Attaching the valves to a plastic plate makes them easier to open and close. Attaching the plastic plate to a styrofoam block stabilizes the plate and valve to prevent unnecessary movement.

10. An insufficient pressure difference between the inlet and outlet of the device can cause spheroids to fall out of the chambers. The minimal height needed to maintain a sufficient pressure difference is 11 in..

11. HEPES-buffered medium is used in device experiments primarily because it can maintain a pH of 7.5 under varying concentrations of carbon dioxide.

12. Opening and closing valves and repeatedly increasing and decreasing the medium flow rate can remove stubborn air bubbles.

13. LS174T cell are used because they readily form spheroids. Any cell line can be used that is sufficiently cohesive to aggregate into distinct cell masses.

14. Positioning the pipette slightly off center insures that the drops are formed at the center the circles.

15. The incubation time for hanging drops and spheroids in PMMA-coated flasks can vary from 3 to 5 days depending on cell growth rate. The time should be adjusted to produce final spheroids that are 500 μm in size.

16. We have found that spheroids toward the middle of the well plate are better formed.

17. Selecting spheroids by eye takes practice, but can be done reliably without use of a stereo microscope.

18. Using room-temperature medium decreases the formation of bubbles within the syringe.

19. If spheroids get stuck, (1) gently tap the base and tip of the needle (through the tubing); (2) gently tap the inlet valve

while opening and closing it; (3) gently wiggle the inlet tube at the intersection with the device.

20. Multiple syringes of spheroids can be injected into the same device. If spheroids are lost or are unsatisfactory, they can be pushed through the post filters to clear these chambers. If some chambers have desirable spheroids, close the packing valves for these chambers. Injecting another syringe gently may allow the remaining chambers to be filled without damaging the already packed chambers.

21. Closing the main outlet valve and opening the packing outlet valves can force spheroids into chambers if they appear to be falling out while changing syringes or while opening the main outlet valve.

22. The typical duration for bacterial administration is 1 h. This is similar to the clearance time in mice. However, this time can be varied to suit the desired protocol.

23. Using 10× magnification we find that a 1000 μm chamber requires two images side-by-side.

24. Different time intervals are used for different applications. We have used less than 1 s intervals to capture fast events and as long as 1 h for long, multiple-day studies.

Acknowledgements

We gratefully acknowledge financial support from the National Science Foundation (Grant No. 1159689) and the National Institutes of Health (Grant No. R01CA120825).

References

1. Toley BJ, Forbes NS (2012) Motility is critical for effective distribution and accumulation of bacteria in tumor tissue. Integr Biol 4:165–176

2. Forbes NS (2010) Engineering the perfect (bacterial) cancer therapy. Nat Rev Cancer 10:785–794

3. Forbes NS, Munn LL, Fukumura D, Jain RK (2003) Sparse initial entrapment of systemically injected Salmonella typhimurium leads to heterogeneous accumulation within tumors. Cancer Res 63:5188–5193

4. Ganai S, Arenas RB, Sauer JP, Bentley B, Forbes NS (2011) In tumors Salmonella migrate away from vasculature toward the transition zone and induce apoptosis. Cancer Gene Ther 18:457–466

5. Ganai S, Arenas RB, Forbes NS (2009) Tumour-targeted delivery of TRAIL using Salmonella typhimurium enhances breast cancer survival in mice. Br J Cancer 101:1683–1691

6. St Jean AT, Zhang M, Forbes NS (2008) Bacterial therapies: completing the cancer treatment toolbox. Curr Opin Biotechnol 19:511–517

7. Walsh CL, Babin BM, Kasinskas RW, Foster JA, McGarry MJ, Forbes NS (2009) A multipurpose microfluidic device designed to mimic microenvironment gradients and develop targeted cancer therapeutics. Lab Chip 9:545–554

8. Toley BJ, Ganz DE, Walsh CL, Forbes NS (2011) Microfluidic device for recreating a tumor microenvironment. J Vis Exp. doi:10.3791/2425

9. Kasinskas RW, Forbes NS (2006) Salmonella typhimurium specifically chemotax and proliferate in heterogeneous tumor tissue in vitro. Biotechnol Bioeng 94:710–721

10. Kasinskas RW, Forbes NS (2007) Salmonella typhimurium lacking ribose chemoreceptors localize in tumor quiescence and induce apoptosis. Cancer Res 67:3201–3209

11. Hong JW, Song S, Shin JH (2013) A novel microfluidic co-culture system for investigation of bacterial cancer targeting. Lab Chip 13(15):3033–3040

12. Elliott N, Lee T, You L, Yuan F (2011) Proliferation behavior of E. coli in a three-dimensional in vitro tumor model. Integr Biol 3:696–705

Chapter 5

Tumor-Targeting Therapy Using Gene-Engineered Anaerobic-Nonpathogenic *Bifidobacterium longum*

Shun'ichiro Taniguchi, Yuko Shimatani, and Minoru Fujimori

Abstract

Despite great progress in molecular-targeting drugs for cancer treatment, there are problems of disease recurrence due to cancer-cell resistance to those drugs, derived from the heterogeneity of tumors. On one hand, the low-oxygen microenvironment present in malignant tumor tissues has been regarded as a source of resistance of cancer cells against conventional therapie, such as radiation and chemotherapy. To overcome these problems, we have been developing a system to selectively deliver a large amount of anticancer drugs to malignant tumors by making use of the limiting factor, hypoxia, in tumors. Our strategy is to use hypoxia as a selective target. Here, we show methods and protocols using the nonpathogenic obligate anaerobic *Bifidobacterium longum* as a drug-delivery system (DDS) to target anaerobic tumor tissue.

Key words Tumor targeting, Cancer therapy, Anaerobic, Oxygen, Hypoxia, Carrier, DDS, Nonpathogenic, *Bifidobacterium longum*

1 Introduction

The usual methods to treat solid malignant tumors are surgery, radiation therapy, and chemotherapy. However, they have not always provided satisfactory results. This is attributed mainly to the existence of metastases and/or acquired resistance of cancer cells to anti-cancer reagents. These recalcitrant problems have led to novel therapeutic methods, including gene therapy, new chemotherapeutic drugs, and recent molecular targeting therapies. Nevertheless, improvements are still needed for novel therapies to overcome cancer-cell drug resistance caused by heterogenic cancer-cell populations within tumors, and also to reduce side effects. To cope with such circumstances, we have tried to selectively target tumors with the obligate anaerobic *Bifidobacterium*, by taking advantage of the anaerobic environment of solid malignant tumors [1, 2] (Fig. 1). The hypoxic environment in malignant tumors is in part due to blood vessels in cancer tissues which are generally

Robert M. Hoffman (ed.), *Bacterial Therapy of Cancer: Methods and Protocols*, Methods in Molecular Biology, vol. 1409, DOI 10.1007/978-1-4939-3515-4_5, © Springer Science+Business Media New York 2016

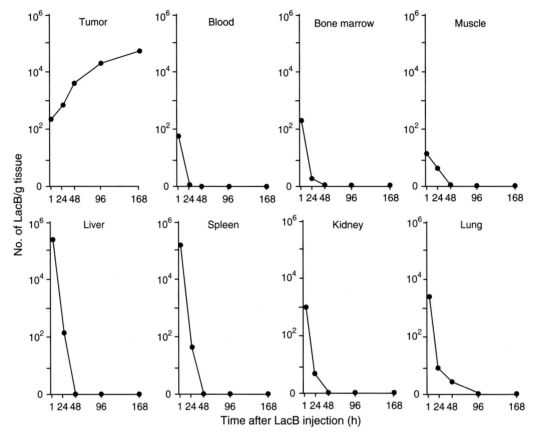

Fig. 1 Specific distribution of *Bifidobacterium bifidum* (Lac B) in tumor tissues following a single i.v. injection of 5×10^6 viable bacilli into Ehrlich solid-tumor-bearing mice. Each point represents the mean of the number of bacilli per gram tissue of eight mice [1]

disorganized with numerous intravascular connections and shunts, and thus unable to deliver fresh blood to the distal regions of malignant tumors [3]. Solid-tumor hypoxia, which is believed to be a causative factor of tumor-cell resistance to radiation therapy and chemotherapy, has recently been attracting attention as a necessary condition for malignant progression [4]. By taking advantage of the anaerobic environment in tumor tissues, we have been developing a delivery system using nonpathogenic anaerobic bacteria, derived from the human intestine [2, 5–8].

The nuance of the word "bacteria" tends to remind people of notions of something dangerous and pathogenic, even when the bacteria are nonpathogenic. The obligate anaerobic bacterium *Bifidobacterium longum* (*BL*) is known not to produce toxic substances. However, bacterial injection in blood has been regarded as dangerous. Common sense dictates that we should not induce artificial bacteremia or septicemia. However, we have repeatedly demonstrated that treatment of solid cancer with *BL* is safe, rational, and effective. We have begun a Phase 1 clinical study through an

Investigational New Drug (IND) application from the Food and Drug Administration (FDA) based on our treatment protocol and chemistry, manufacturing, and control (CMC) and good manufacturing practice (GMP) of our bacterial. A recent review article described the possibility of cancer treatment with bacteria and highlighted the potential utility of bacteria therapy of cancer using genetic engineering [9].

Human life is dependent on co-existence with microorganisms. Intestinal bacteria are one such example. Genetic engineering techniques have been providing recombinant medicines through bacteria and plasmids. The recent emergence of probiotics has shown potential not only for intestinal disorders, but also for care of the skin and oral cavity [10, 11]. Our Phase I trial is to expand the utility of probiotics to systemically treat solid cancers using intravenous administration of anaerobic *Bifidobacterium longum*.

In addition to our Phase I trial, Phase I trials in the USA of attenuated *Salmonella typhimurium* and *Clostridium* to treat solid cancers have been performed [12, 13].

In the present report, the authors describe their Materials and Methods and their findings to demonstrate potential use of *Bifidobacterium longum* for systemic delivery to treat anaerobic solid tumors (Fig. 1).

2   Materials

Sprague-Dawley rats (Japan SLC, Hamamatsu, Japan).

Standard rodent diet (Oriental Yeast, Tokyo, Japan).

C57BL/6 mice (Japan SLC).

BALB/c-nu/nu mice.

DMBA (Yasuda Pharmacy, Maebashi, Japan).

MRMT-1 rat mammary gland carcinoma cells (Cell Resource Center for Biomedical Research, Tohoku University, Sendai, Japan).

RPMI-1640 (Sigma, St. Louis, MO, USA).

B16-F10 melanoma cells.

Lewis lung cancer cells.

Dulbecco's modified Eagle's medium.

B. longum 105-A (Dr. Mitsuoka).

Plasmid pBLES100-S-eCD.

Gene Pulser apparatus (Bio-Rad Laboratories, Hercules, CA).

Anaerobic jars (Mitsubishi Gas Chemical, Tokyo, Japan).

MRS agar plates (Oxoid, Basingstoke, UK).

Rabbit anti-CD polyclonal antibody (Sawady Technology, Tokyo, Japan).

GS/MS (GS: HP6890, MSD: HP5973, Column: HP-50+; Hewlett Packard).

Dunkin Hartley guinea pigs.

3   Methods and Protocols [5–8]

3.1   Animals

1. For an autochthonous tumor system, female, 6-week-old Sprague-Dawley rats were used in the present study. Rats were fed a standard rodent diet in the Shinshu University animal center (Matsumoto, Japan) (*see* **Note 1**).

2. The animal experiments in this study were carried out in accordance with the Guidelines for Animal Experimentation of the Shinshu University School of Medicine.

3. For a syngeneic transplantable tumor system, male C57BL/6 mice, 6–8 weeks, were used in the study.

4. Mice were fed a standard rodent diet in the Shinshu University animal center.

5. For a human tumor system, immune-deficient BALB/c*nu/nu* mice were used.

3.2   Tumors

1. As the autochthonous tumor source, rats were given 10 mg of DMBA in 1 mL sesame oil by intragastric gavage once weekly for 2 weeks. Twenty-three weeks after the first dose of DMBA, 89 % of the rats developed autochthonous mammary tumors. For each tumor, the maximum diameter (A), diameter at right angles to A (B), and thickness (C) were measured using sliding calipers. Tumor volume was estimated as $1/2 \times A \times B \times C$ (*see* **Note 1**).

2. As the source of transplanted tumors, MRMT-1 rat mammary gland carcinoma cells were cultured in medium containing RPMI-1640 and 10 % fetal bovine serum (heat inactivated), at 37 °C in an atmosphere of 5 % CO_2. A total of 5×10^6 cancer cells were inoculated into the dorsal skin of rats. Solid tumors were obtained 2 weeks after inoculation.

3. For the mouse tumor system, B16-F10 melanoma cells and Lewis lung cancer cells were maintained as monolayer cultures in Dulbecco's modified Eagle's medium supplemented with 10 % fetal bovine serum at 37 °C in an atmosphere of 5 % CO_2.

4. A total of 5×10^5 cancer cells were inoculated into the right thigh muscle of male C57BL/6 mice. Solid tumors obtained 2 weeks after inoculation were then used for the present study.

5. For the human tumor system, human breast cancer, stomach cancer, and colon cancer cells were used (*see* **Notes 2** and **3**).

3.3 Bacteria

B. longum 105-A, obtained from Dr. Mitsuoka, was anaerobically cultured at 37 °C to middle log phase in modified Briggs broth using 2 % lactose instead of glucose.

3.4 Plasmid Construction

1. A plasmid, pBLES100-S-eCD, comprising the HU gene promoter and the cytosine deaminase gene in the shuttle vector pBLES100, was constructed as described by Nakamura et al. [6].

2. The HU gene that encodes a histone-like DNA-binding protein is expressed at high levels in *B. longum* [14].

3. The CD gene was ligated to the HU gene promoter and then inserted into pBLES100 to form pBLES100-S-eCD.

3.5 Transformation of Bifidobacterium longum with pBLES100- S-eCD

1. The pBLES100-S-eCD plasmid was transferred directly into *B. longum* 105-A by electroporation with a Gene Pulser apparatus (inter-electrode distance, 0.2 cm) (*see* **Note 4**).

2. Electroporation was performed at 2.0 kV and a 25 μF capacitor setting with the pulse controller set at 200 Ω parallel resistance, yielding a pulse duration of 4.1–4.5 ms.

3. Stable transformants were obtained with an efficiency of 1.6×10^4 transformants/μg DNA under optimum conditions.

4. Transformed *B. longum* (*B. longum*/e-CD) was grown under anaerobic conditions at 37 °C in Briggs broth containing 75 μg/ml spectinomycin (*see* **Note 5**).

3.6 Treatment of Rats with Systemic Administration of Genetically-Engineered Bifidobacterium longum

1. Eleven rats bearing chemically-induced mammary tumors received 5×10^8 CFU/day of *B. longum*/e-CD via tail vein injection for 4 days.

2. The total amount of *B. longum*/e-CD injected was 2×10^9 CFU/rat. Rats were given 500 mg/kg/day of 5-FC by intragastric gavage from 4 days after final injection of *B. longum*/e-CD. 5-FC was given daily for 72 days.

3. The tumor size in the injected group ($n=11$) was compared with that in the non-injected group ($n=5$) (Fig. 2).

4. Treatment of human tumors grown in immunodeficient *nu/nu* mice was carried out in a similar way as the rat system and anti-tumor efficacy was observed (Fig. 3).

3.7 Detection of B. longum in Various Tissues

1. Seven rats bearing MRMT-1 mammary gland carcinoma received 3.6×10^9 CFU/day of *B. longum*/e-CD through the tail vein for 3 days, and thereafter were given 5-FC at 500 mg/kg/day by intragastric gavage from 4 days after the final injection of bacteria until the day they were sacrificed.

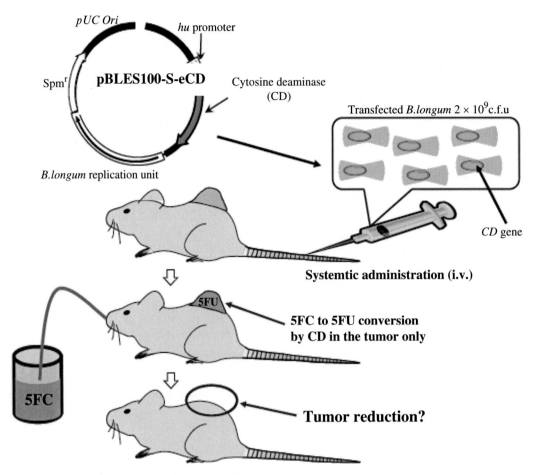

Fig. 2 Concept of cancer treatment by combining *Escherichia coli* cytosine deaminase (e-CD)-transformed *Bifidobacterium longum* (*B. longum*/e-CD) (i.v.) with the prodrug 5-fluorocytosine (5-FC) (given daily) which is converted to 5-fluorouracil (5-FU) [2]

2. All rats were euthanized on day 7 after 5-FC had been given.

3. Normal tissues (liver, heart, lung, and kidney) and tumor tissues were obtained for detection of *B. longum* in various tissues.

4. Normal tissues and tumors were excised and minced thoroughly, and samples were weighed and homogenized with anaerobic diluent.

5. The diluted tissue homogenates were spread in duplicate at 200 μL on MRS agar plates containing spectinomycin.

6. All plates were placed in anaerobic jars at 37 °C under anaerobic conditions.

7. On day 3 of culture, the number of colonies per plate was determined. In addition, tumors and livers were fixed in 10 % formalin solution, sectioned in paraffin, and treated with Gram's stain.

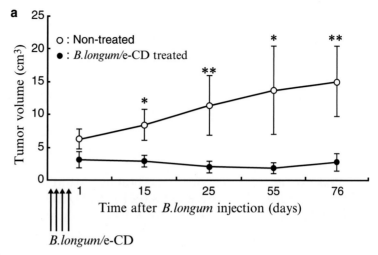

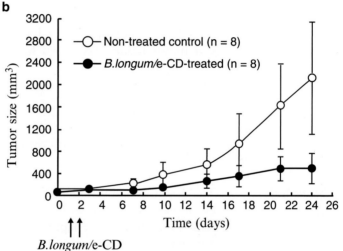

Fig. 3 Anti-tumor efficacy of i.v.-injected genetically-engineered *B. longum/e*-CD to express *Escherichia coli* cytosine deaminase (e-CD) combined with 5-fluorocytosine (5-FC) (given orally). (**a**) Comparison of tumor volumes of non-injected rats (*n* = 5) with those of *B. longum/e*-CD i.v.-injected rats (*n* = 15). Rats bearing 7,12-dimethylbenz(a)anthracene-induced mammary tumors received i.v. *B. longum/e*-CD and 500 mg/kg/day of 5-FC. *$P < 0.05$; **$P < 0.01$. (**b**) Anti-tumor efficacy of *B. longum/e*-CD in nude mice transplanted with KPL-1 human mammary tumor cells. Tumor-bearing nude mice (*n* = 8) were given a dose of transformed bacteria cells i.v. (5.9×10^9 CFU/mouse), followed by 5-FC (orally) for 21 days (cited from ref. 2)

3.8 Immunohisto-chemistry

1. Serial sections of tumor tissues were treated with Gram's stain to detect the presence of *B. longum*/pBLES100-S-eCD and with rabbit anti-CD polyclonal antibody to confirm CD expression of *B. longum*/pBLES100-S-eCD in the tumor tissue.

2. MRMT-1 mammary-gland carcinoma-bearing rats were euthanized 11 days after *B. longum*/pBLES100-S-eCD

injection. Tumors were then excised, fixed in 10 % formalin solution, sectioned in paraffin, and immunostained for CD with the avidin–biotin complex method using a rabbit anti-CD polyclonal antibody diluted 1:800. Immunoreactivity was visualized with DAB. As a control, some sections were stained using normal rabbit serum instead of rabbit anti-CD polyclonal antibody.

3. In the tumor tissues, the serial section immunostained for CD was treated with Gram's stain [8].

3.9 Measurement of 5-FC Concentration in Various Tissues

1. Nine rats bearing MRMT-1 mammary gland carcinoma received 3.6×10^9 CFU/day of *B. longum*/e-CD through the tail vein for 3 days, and thereafter were given 5-FC at 500 mg/kg/day by intragastric gavage for 4 days after the final injection of bacteria.

2. All rats were euthanized on day 4 after 5-FC had been administered. Normal tissues (liver, lung, heart, spleen, and kidney) and tumor tissues were used for the measurement of 5-FC concentration by GS/MS (GS: HP6890, MSD: HP5973, Column: HP-50+; Hewlett Packard).

3. A rat given 5-FC without injection of *B. longum*/e-CD was used as a control.

4. The tumor-specific production of 5-FU was observed [8] (Fig. 4).

3.10 Antigenic Test

1. The systemic immunogenicity of *B. longum*/pBLES100-S-eCD was evaluated with the active systemic anaphylaxis (ASA) reaction. The anaphylactic activity of IgG was evaluated with the passive cutaneous anaphylaxis (PCA) reaction in guinea pigs.

2. For sensitization of guinea pigs, 2×10^9 CFU *B. longum*/pBLES100-S-eCD diluted with physiological saline (saline) and mixed with Freund's complete adjuvant (FCA), equivalently or not, was injected subcutaneously into the dorsal skin of male Dunkin Hartley guinea pigs at the time of antigen challenge (once weekly for 3 weeks).

3. As a positive control, 0.5 % OVA (ovalbumin) diluted with saline and mixed with an equal volume of FCA was used. Saline mixed with an equal volume of FCA was used as the negative control. In the ASA reaction, the actively-immunized guinea pigs were injected intravenously with *B. longum*/e-CD or OVA 14 days after final sensitization.

4. Anaphylaxis symptoms were quantified by the following criterion: (−) no symptom; (±) scrub of face or ear and/or

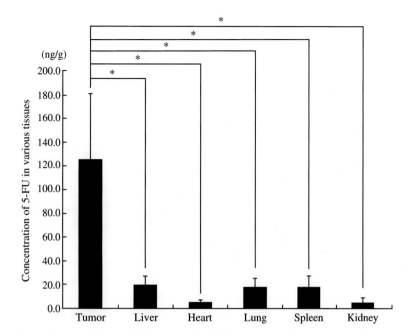

Fig. 4 Measurement of 5-fluorouracil (5-FU) concentration in various tissues. Tissue distribution of 5-FU in rats bearing MRMT-1 mammary gland carcinoma. Rats were given *Bifidobacterium longum*/eCD at 1.1×10^{10} CFU/rat i.v., and 5-fluorocytosine (5-FC) by intragastric gavage for 4 days starting from 4 days after bacterial injection. The concentration of 5-FU in normal tissues (liver, heart, lung, spleen, and kidney) and tumor tissues was measured. A rat given 5-FC without injection of *B. longum*/e-CD was used as a control. The 5-FU concentrations in bacteria-injected rats were adjusted by subtraction of the 5-FU value of the control rat as the background value. *$P < 0.05$ (cited from ref. 2)

scratch of nose; (+) coughing or locomotion ataxia; (++) convulsion or roll, but no death observed within 1 h; (+++) death observed within 1 h. In the PCA reaction, immunized guinea pigs were sacrificed and blood samples were collected 14 days after final sensitization to obtain antiserum from each guinea pig.

5. Normal guinea pigs were shaved and 0.05 mL of each serum dilution was injected intradermally into the dorsal skin. After 4 h, the animals were injected intravenously with 1 mL antigen (*B. longum*/e-CD or OVA) and 0.5 mL 1 % Evans blue solution.

6. After 30 min, the animals were killed, the dorsal skin was peeled off, and blue spots within the intradermal sites were measured. A PCA reaction was judged to be positive when the blue spot measured more than 5 mm².

7. No significant reaction was observed in either the ASA or the PCA reaction [8].

8. In further tests to examine immunological toxicity, the blood levels of various inflammatory cytokines, such as interleukin (IL-1β, IL-18, and IL-6), were examined after i.v. injection of *B. longum* carrying the e-CD expression vector [2] (*see* **Note 6**).

4   Notes

1. Generally, an autochthonous tumor system is relatively difficult to cure compared with a transplanted tumor system, since the tumor is comprised of cells which have escaped from host immune surveillance.

2. When tumor cells were transplanted into animals, the number of cells should be as small as possible to mimic a human tumor system where one nodule is produced from single or a few cancer cells. In such tumors, *Bifidobacterium longum* can localize even in a small tumor.

3. To assay pre-clinical anti-tumor activity, we used allogenic transplantation of human cancer cells into immune-deficient nude mice. Even in the immune-deficient system, the *Bifidobacterium longum* was safely administered without a severe infusion reaction as long as the i.v. injection speed was low.

4. The expression vector, pBLES100-S-eCD, was later modified by introducing a point mutation into the active site (D314A) of eCD. Consequently, the affinity of mutated eCD to natural cytosine was decreased but relatively increased against 5-FC, leading to enhancement of the production of 5-FU to the level of 1 μg/g tumor tissue after systemic injection of the gene-engineered *Bifidobacterium longum*. Even under these conditions, the production of 5-FU was marginally detected in other organs because the bacteria did not localize in normal tissues.

5. The recipient, *Bifidobacterium longum* 105A, was made 5-FU resistant.

6. No inflammatory cytokines were induced by inoculation of *B. longum*, whereas *E. coli* clearly induced cytokines such as interleukin (IL)-1β, IL-18, and IL-6. These results indicated that genetically-modified *B. longum* does not induce septicemia (Fig. 5).

To evaluate the toxicity of genetically-modified *B. longum*, a number of preclinical studies have also been carried out in several animal species, including normal mice, nude mice, normal rats,

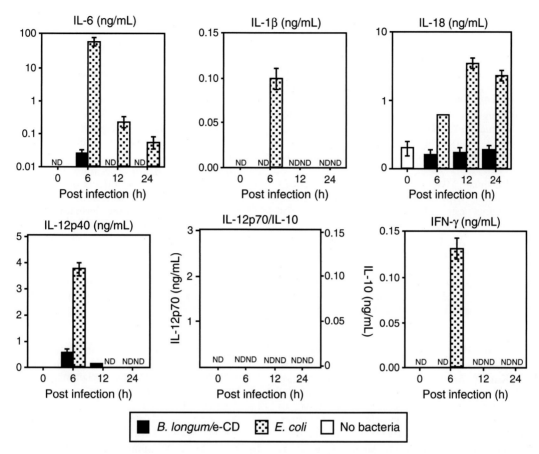

Fig. 5 Production of inflammatory cytokines in C57BL/6 mice infected i.v. with *Escherichia coli* cytosine deaminase (e-CD)-transformed *Bifidobacterium longum* (*B. longum*/e-CD) or nonpathogenic *E. coli* (control). Cytokines were assessed with ELISA 6 h after infection. *Closed bars*, blood of mice injected with *B. longum*/e-CD; *dotted bars*, blood of mice injected with nonpathogenic *E. coli*; *open bars*, normal blood. *IFN* interferon, *IL* interleukin, *ND* not detected (cited from ref. 2)

nude rats, and monkeys. Both pharmacological and preliminary general toxicity studies were performed, none of which revealed serious toxicities.

Acknowledgement

We thank all of our colleagues at Anaeropharma Science, Inc. for their technical support and useful discussions.

References

1. Kimura NT, Taniguchi S, Aoki K, Baba T (1980) Selective localization and growth of *Bifidobacterium bifidom* in mouse tumors following intraveneous administration. Cancer Res 40:2061–2068

2. Taniguchi S, Fujimori M, Sasaki T, Tsutsui H, Shimatani Y, Seki K, Amano J (2010) Targeting solid tumors with non-pathogenic obligate anaerobic bacteria. Cancer Sci 101:1925–1932

3. Dewhirst MW, Cao Y, Moeller B (2008) Cycling hypoxia and free radicals regulate angiogenesis and radiotherapy response. Nat Rev Cancer 8:425–437

4. Sullivan R, Graham CH (2007) Hypoxia-driven selection of the metastatic phenotype. Cancer Metastasis Rev 26:319–331

5. Yazawa K, Fujimori M, Nakamura T, Sasaki T, Amano J, Kano Y, Taniguchi S (2001) *Bifidobacterium longum* as a delivery system for gene therapy of chemically induced rat mammary tumors. Breast Cancer Res Treat 66:165–170

6. Nakamura T, Sasaki T, Fujimori M, Yazawa K, Kano Y, Amano J, Taniguchi S (2002) Cloned cytosine deaminase gene expression of *Bifidobacterium longum* and application to enzyme/pro-drug therapy of hypoxic solid tumors. Biosci Biotechnol Biochem 66:2362–2366

7. Yazawa K, Fujimori M, Amano J, Kano Y, Taniguchi S (2000) *Bifidobacterium longum* as a delivery system for cancer gene therapy: selective localization and growth in hypoxic tumors. Cancer Gene Ther 7:269–274

8. Sasaki T, Fujimori M, Hamaji Y, Hama Y, Ito K, Amano J, Taniguchi S (2006) Genetically engineered Bifidobacterium longum for tumor-targeting enzyme-prodrug therapy of autochthonous mammary tumors in rats. Cancer Sci 97:649–657

9. Forbes NS (2010) Engineering the perfect (bacterial) cancer therapy. Nat Rev Cancer 10:785–794

10. Gueniche A, Knaudt B, Schuck E, Volz T, Bastien P et al (2008) Effects of nonpathogenic gramnegative bacterium Vitreoscilla filiformis lysate on atopic dermatitis: a prospective, randomized, double-blind, placebo-controlled clinical study. Br J Dermatol 159:1357–1363

11. He X, Lux R, Kuramitsu HK, Anderson MH, Shi W (2009) Achieving probiotic effects via modulating oral microbial ecology. Adv Dent Res 21:53–56

12. Toso JF, Gill VJ, Hwu P, Marincola FM, Restifo NP, Schwartzentruber DJ et al (2002) Phase I study of the intravenous administration of attenuated Salmonella typhimurium to patients with metastatic melanoma. J Clin Oncol 20:142–152

13. Wei MQ, Mengesha A, Good D, Anne J (2008) Bacterial targeted tumour therapy dawn of a new era. Cancer Lett 259:16–27

14. Takeuchi A, Matsumura H, Kano Y (2002) Cloning and expression in *Escherichia coli* of a gene, *hup*, encoding the histone-like protein HU of *Bifidobacterium longum*. Biosci Biotechnol Biochem 66:598–603

Chapter 6

Noninvasive In Vivo Imaging to Follow Bacteria Engaged in Cancer Therapy

Sara Leschner and Siegfried Weiss

Abstract

Non-invasive in vivo imaging represents a powerful tool to monitor cellular and molecular processes in the living animal. In the special case of bacteria-mediated cancer therapy using bioluminescent bacteria, it opens up the possibility to follow the course of the microorganisms into the tumor via the circulation. The mechanism by which bacteria elicit their anti-tumor potential is not completely understood. However, this knowledge is crucial to improve bacteria as an anti-cancer tool that can be introduced into the clinic. For the study of these aspects, in vivo imaging can be considered a key technology.

Key words In vivo imaging, Luminescent bacteria, Lux operon, Firefly luciferase, Chromosomal integration

1 Introduction

In vivo imaging with bioluminescent bacteria can be used to monitor infections in tumor-bearing mice [1]. This method has convincing advantages over conventional means to track bacterial locations in mice, such as plating of organ homogenates to determine colony-forming units (CFU). Concerning reliability and validity, in vivo imaging is outstanding as it allows following the infection process in individual mice at consecutive time points. Sacrificing the animals for analysis is obviously not required. As a consequence, fewer mice are needed for an experiment. First, this is generally desirable in order to reduce the number of experimental animals for animal welfare. Second, this renders studies more cost-and labor-efficient.

As a prerequisite to study bacterial infections in an in vivo imaging system, a reporter strain has to be available. Depending on the demand of the experiment, a reporter strain can be simply purchased or acquired from colleagues, if possible. However, for specific needs such as in bacteria-mediated cancer therapy variants are required that are not commonly used. Thus, the strain might have to be newly constructed. Various expression plasmids can be used

Robert M. Hoffman (ed.), *Bacterial Therapy of Cancer: Methods and Protocols*, Methods in Molecular Biology, vol. 1409, DOI 10.1007/978-1-4939-3515-4_6, © Springer Science+Business Media New York 2016

for this purpose. However, high-copy-number plasmids, e.g., with a Puc origin of replication (ori), are not advisable. Although these vectors should give extremely bright signals, such plasmids have the tendency to be lost quickly from the transformants in vivo when antibiotic selection for plasmid maintenance is no longer possible. This is most likely due to the extreme metabolic burden such expression plasmids present for the bacteria. Low-copy-number plasmids such as pSC101 would result in more stable transformants. However, eventually, such reporter-encoding expression plasmids might also be lost. Since this is a random event, it is not predictable whether the loss occurs early during colonization or late. This renders a serious quantitative experiment difficult. A way around this problem would be to introduce balanced suicide plasmids where the plasmid complements a chromosomal deletion of a gene encoding an essential metabolic enzyme. However, to us the stable integration of the expression cassette into the bacterial chromosome appears to be the better alternative. For chromosomal integration, we targeted the transposon 7 (Tn7) attachment site, which can be found in *E. coli* and *S. typhimurium* as well as in other Gram-negative bacteria. This targeted integration ensures that we do not disrupt any essential gene. How this is achieved is the scope of the present article.

The principle of the Tn7 integration of constructs into the bacterial chromosome is as follows: Including the recipient bacterial strain, three strains are needed for this method (Fig. 1). The carrier strain contains a plasmid with the desired construct located between the two Tn7 recognition sites Tn7L and Tn7R. This plasmid has a pir-dependent ori and therefore has to be transformed into a strain supplying the pir product of the lysogenic bacteriophage λ, such as SM10λpir. The same holds true for the helper strain which provides the transposase required to catalyze the integration step on a pir-dependent plasmid. Both plasmids contain mobilization elements in addition. Once all three strains are mixed and placed on a membrane filter, the helper and carrier strain will conjugate with the recipient and transfer their plasmids. As these plasmids are both pir dependent, they cannot be propagated in the recipient strain. However, the construct might integrate into the bacterial chromosome via homologous recombination of the Tn7 recognition sites catalyzed by the transposase. Successful integration events can be detected by antibiotic selection. Positive clones should now be resistant to kanamycin but no longer to ampicillin, since this marker is only carried by plasmids and will be lost.

Various bioluminescent reporter genes exist that can be used for noninvasive in vivo imaging. Fluorescent proteins (photoluminescence) as well as chemiluminescent enzymes such as bacterial lux or insect luciferases are available. In this chapter, the stable use of a lux operon and the firefly luciferase are introduced.

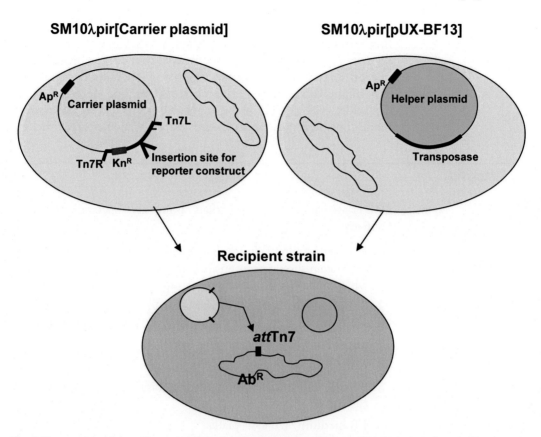

Fig. 1 Chromosomal integration using the mini-Tn7 transposon. Successful integration of a specific construct requires three strains: SM10λpir containing the carrier plasmid with the construct flanked by the Tn7 recognition sites (Tn7L and Tn7R); a helper strain in which the plasmid supplies the transposase necessary to integrate into the chromosome of the third, namely, the recipient strain. Upon mixing all three strains, conjugation of carrier and helper strains takes place toward the recipient bacterium. Both plasmids possess mobilization elements which allow them to enter the recipient strain. Once inside the bacterial cell, the transposase catalyzes the integration of the transposon into the recipient's *att*Tn7 (chromosomal Tn7 attachment site)

Various bacteria produce light using the so-called lux operon (*luxCDABE*) such as *Photorhabdus luminescens*, a pathogen of nematodes. In this system, *LuxCDE* encodes a fatty-acid reductase complex that is involved in synthesis of fatty aldehydes for the luminescence reaction. This reaction is catalyzed by the luciferase LuxA and LuxB subunits [2]. Therefore, all components that are required for the enzymatic reaction to produce light are already present in bacteria expressing the *lux* operon. This renders the addition of a substrate (such as luciferin in the case of the luciferase system) unnecessary which represents a big advantage concerning convenience of the experimental process and cost reduction. Using the firefly luciferase *luc*, introduced in this chapter as an example, requires luciferin injections into the mice prior to imaging [3]. As the substrate is degraded within the body of the mouse, additional injections might be required for later time points of image acquisition. However, the advantage of the firefly luciferase systems is the superior strength of the signal compared to the signal from the *lux* operon. In a case of a weak expression or a low number of bacteria, this might determine whether a signal can be detected at all. Therefore, the choice of the reporter system has to be carefully made considering the special needs of the particular experiment.

2   Materials

(Materials or methods marked bold are specific for firefly luciferase).

2.1   Construction of Reporter Strain via Chromosomal Integration

1. Recipient strain of choice that should be used for in vivo imaging (this strain should carry an antibiotic resistance gene for selection which must not be kanamycin or ampicillin—*see* **Note 1**).
2. SM10λpir[pUX-BF5] (carrier strain) [4].
3. Plasmid containing the lux operon or the *luc* gene (e.g., plite201) under control of a constitutive or inducible promoter.
4. Chemically-competent SM10λpir.
5. Suitable enzymes to clone the promoter lux/*luc* construct into the carrier plasmid.
6. LB medium/LB agar plates.
7. Antibiotics: kanamycin and ampicillin.
8. 0.45 μm nitrocellulose membrane filter.

2.2   Cancer-Cell Inoculation

1. Cancer cell line of choice.
2. Cell culture medium.
3. TE (trypsin: 0.5 g/ml, EDTA in PBS: 0.2 g/ml).
4. PBS.
5. Insulin syringes.
6. Appropriate recipient mouse strain syngeneic with the cancer cell line.

2.3   Preparation of the Inoculum

1. Reporter strain.
2. LB medium supplemented with the appropriate antibiotics.
3. PBS.

2.4   In Vivo Imaging

1. In vivo imaging system such as IVIS 200 from PerkinElmer.
2. Inoculum of the reporter strain.
3. Tumor-bearing mouse.
4. Insulin syringe.

5. Isoflurane or other anesthesia.

6. **Luciferin (150 mg/kg from Synchem or PerkinElmer).**

3 Methods

3.1 Construction of Reporter Strain via Chromosomal Integration

1. Carrier plasmid containing construct of choice using the backbone of plasmid pUX-BF5 [4]. The reporter construct has to be placed in between the two transposon attachment sites Tn7R and Tn7L without interfering with the kanamycin-resistance gene (Fig. 1).

2. Once the carrier plasmid has been constructed and propagated in SM10λpir, prepare overnight cultures of all required strains (recipient strain, carrier, and helper strain) in LB medium supplemented with the appropriate antibiotics. Note that SM10λpir strains have to be incubated at 28 °C in order to prevent induction of the bacteriophage (*see* **Note 2**).

3. Grow bacterial cultures to an OD_{600} of approximately 1.0.

4. Mix 500 μl of each culture in a reaction tube and centrifuge at $3500 \times g$ for 5 min.

5. Discard supernatant and resuspend the pellet in 1 ml LB without antibiotics.

6. Centrifuge again at $3500 \times g$ for 5 min.

7. Discard supernatant and resuspend the pellet in 20 μl LB medium without antibiotics.

8. Sterilely place a 0.45 μm nitrocellulose membrane filter on an LB plate without antibiotics.

9. Carefully pipet the resuspended culture mixture on the filter and allow to dry for 5 min.

10. Incubate the plate inverted at 28 °C for 24–30 h.

11. Take the filter from the plate with a sterile forceps, place it in a reaction tube, and add 1 ml LB medium.

12. Vortex gently for 10 s.

13. Plate 100 μl on one and the residual 900 μl on another LB plate containing 30 μg/ml kanamycin and the antibiotic that the recipient strain carries as a selection marker and incubate overnight at 37 °C.

14. Pick single colonies and streak them out on LB plates containing 100 μg/ml ampicillin as well as on LB plates containing 30 μg/ml kanamycin and the antibiotic the recipient is resistant to.

15. After overnight incubation at 37 °C, clones that have successfully integrated the reporter construct should grow on kanamycin-, but not on ampicillin-containing plates.

3.2 Cancer Cell Inoculation

1. Grow cancer cells at 37 °C and 5 % CO_2 in a humidified atmosphere.

2. Detach adherent cells by incubating with TE for 5 min at 37 °C or use a cell scraper.

3. Centrifuge the cell suspension for 5 min at $250 \times g$ at 4 °C.

4. Discard the supernatant and resuspend the pellet in ice-cold PBS.

5. Adjust cell suspension to an appropriate cell number per ml.

6. Inject 100 µl of this cell suspension subcutaneously into the recipient mouse.

7. Allow the tumor to grow to a volume of approximately 200 mm^3.

3.3 Preparation of the Inoculum

1. Prepare an overnight LB culture with appropriate antibiotics for the reporter strain to grow at 37 °C while shaking.

2. Dilute the overnight culture 1:300 in fresh medium and incubate at 37 °C, with shaking to achieve an OD_{600} of 0.2–0.4.

3. Centrifuge the culture at $3500 \times g$ for 5 min at room temperature.

4. Discard the supernatant and resuspend the pellet in PBS.

5. Repeat this washing step twice.

6. Adjust the OD_{600} of the washed culture to an appropriate inoculation dose.

3.4 In Vivo Image Acquisition

1. Infect the tumor-bearing mice with the previously prepared inoculum by the desired route.

2. Five minutes before imaging, inject mice intravenously or intraperitoneally with luciferin.

3. Anesthetize the mice and place them into the IVIS imager, carefully making sure the mouse nose is firmly attached into the nose cone to ensure oxygen and anesthesia supply.

4. Adjust IVIS settings to "luminescent" and choose correct *field of view* (FOV) according to the number of mice that should be imaged, acquisition time, f-stop, and binning according to the strength of the expected signal.

5. Acquire image (Fig. 2).

4 Notes

1. The recipient bacterial strain should carry an antibiotic-resistance gene. This should NOT be an ampicillin-nor a kanamycin-resistance gene as they are both on the carrier and/or helper plasmid. An antibiotic-resistance gene as a marker of the recipient strain allows selection for clones that have successfully integrated the transposon (Subheading 3.1, **step 13**).

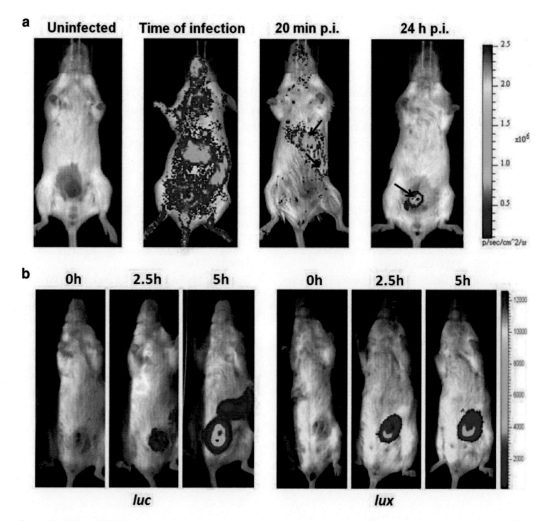

Fig. 2 Bacterial infections with *lux*- and *luc*-carrying *Salmonella typhimurium* in tumor-bearing mice. CT26 tumor-bearing mice were infected with *S. typhimurium* SL7207 carrying different constructs. The *black arrow* points at the subcutaneous tumor growing on the abdomen of the mice. (**a**) Constitutive *lux* expression was used to show *Salmonella* accumulation at the time of intravenous infection, 20 min postinfection (p.i.) and 1 day after infection (reproduced from [1]). (**b**) Inducible expression can be realized using *luc* (*left three panels*), or *lux* (*right three panels*) under control of an l-arabinose promoter [5]. Mice have been infected 3 days before inducing luminescence expression. Induction is achieved by intraperitoneal injection of 120 mg l-arabinose. Images were acquired at the indicated time points (reproduced from [5])

2. All SM10λpir strains have to be propagated at 28 °C in order to prevent induction of the endogenous bacteriophage, the activation of which would result in killing of the bacterial cells. Once the construct is integrated into the chromosome of the recipient, this strain can be grown at 37 °C again.

Acknowledgment

This work was supported in part by grants from the Deutsche Krebshilfe, the German Research Council (DFG), the Ministry for Education and Research (BMBF), the Helmholtz Research School for Infection Research, the Hannover Biomedical Research School (HBRS), and the Centre for Infection Biology (ZIB).

References

1. Leschner S, Westphal K, Dietrich N, Viegas N, Jablonska J, Lyszkiewicz M et al (2009) Tumor invasion of Salmonella enterica serovar Typhimurium is accompanied by strong hemorrhage promoted by TNF-alpha. PLoS One 4:e6692

2. Meighen EA (1991) Molecular biology of bacterial bioluminescence. Microbiol Rev 55:123–142

3. Vieira J, da Pinto SL, Esteves da Silva JC (2012) Advances in the knowledge of light emission by firefly luciferin and oxyluciferin. J Photochem Photobiol B 117:33–39

4. Bao Y, Lies DP, Fu H, Roberts GP (1991) An improved Tn7-based system for the single-copy insertion of cloned genes into chromosomes of gram-negative bacteria. Gene 109:167–168

5. Loessner H, Endmann A, Leschner S, Westphal K, Rohde M, Miloud T et al (2007) Remote control of tumour-targeted Salmonella enterica serovar Typhimurium by the use of l-arabinose as inducer of bacterial gene expression in vivo. Cell Microbiol 9:1529–1537

Chapter 7

In Vivo Bioluminescence Imaging of Intratumoral Bacteria

Michelle Cronin, Ali R. Akin, Kevin P. Francis, and Mark Tangney

Abstract

This chapter describes the use of whole-body bioluminescent imaging (BLI) for the study of bacterial trafficking in live mice, with an emphasis on the use of bacteria in therapy of cancer. Bacteria present an attractive class of vector for cancer therapy, possessing a natural ability to grow preferentially within tumors following systemic administration. Bacteria engineered to express the lux gene cassette permit BLI detection of the bacteria and tumor sites concurrently. The location and levels of bacteria within tumors over time can be readily examined, visualized in two or three dimensions. The method is applicable to a wide range of bacterial species and tumor xenograft types. This article describes the protocol for analysis of bioluminescent bacteria within subcutaneous tumor-bearing mice. This powerful, and inexpensive, real-time imaging strategy represents an ideal method for the study of bacteria in vivo in the context of cancer research. This protocol outlines the procedure for studying lux-tagged *Escherichia coli* and *Bifidobacterium breve* in mice, demonstrating the spatial and temporal readout from 2D and 3D BLI achievable with whole-body *in vivo* luminescence imaging.

Key words *Escherichia coli*, *Bifidobacterium breve*, Bacterial therapy, Gene therapy, Cancer, Vector, Lux, Optical imaging, Luciferase

1 Introduction

The ability to track microbes in real-time in vivo is of enormous value for preclinical investigations [1]. In the context of gene therapy, the use of biological agents for delivery of therapeutic genes to patients has shown great promise [2–4]. Similar to viruses, the innate biological properties of bacteria permit efficient DNA delivery to cells or tissues, particularly in the context of cancer. It has been shown that bacteria are naturally capable of homing to tumors when systemically administered resulting in high levels of replication locally [5]. Tumor-selective bacterial colonization now appears to be both bacterial-species- and tumor-origin-independent, since both anaerobic and aerobic bacteria are capable of colonizing tumors, and furthermore even small tumors lacking an anaerobic center are colonized. Factors such as the irregular, leaky blood supply, hypoxia, local immune suppression, inflammation, and a unique

Robert M. Hoffman (ed.), *Bacterial Therapy of Cancer: Methods and Protocols*, Methods in Molecular Biology, vol. 1409, DOI 10.1007/978-1-4939-3515-4_7, © Springer Science+Business Media New York 2016

nutrient supply (e.g., purines) in tumors have been proposed to play a role [6]. Overall, the precise mechanism(s) behind preferential bacterial tumor colonization remain unknown. We have engineered a number of strains to express the luxABCDE cassette [7–12]. The protocol outlined in this chapter exploits lux-tagged nonpathogenic commensal *Escherichia coli* K-12 MG1655 and *Bifidobacterium breve* UCC2003 as model organisms.

Several studies have outlined the safety of intravenous (iv) administration of non-pathogenic bacterial strains to mice and their ability to grow specifically within tumors [3, 13]. An advantage of using bacterial luciferase is that the *lux* cassette encodes the enzymes required for substrate biosynthesis, resulting in a directly-imageable agent [1]. BLI is based on the detection of bioluminescent light from the subject through the use of a cooled charged-coupled device (CCD) camera. The relatively simple instrumentation and lack of requirement for radioactivity put the technology well within the reach of the average laboratory. BLI displays many benefits when compared with other in vivo modalities. It is easy to use, inexpensive, and rapid. BLI facilitates imaging of multiple animals simultaneously, producing little background with high sensitivity.

This study visualizes the growth of *lux*-labeled bacteria in live tumor-bearing mice, both two and three dimensionally, using in vivo BLI [9]. The nonpathogenic commensal bacteria MG1655 and UCC2003, each expressing the *luxABCDE* operon, were intravenously (iv) administered to mice bearing subcutaneous (s.c.) *FLuc*-expressing xenograft tumors. The bacterial *lux* signal was detected specifically in tumors of mice post-IV administration and bioluminescence correlated with the number of bacteria recovered from tissue. Through whole-body imaging for both *lux* and *FLuc*, bacteria and tumors were co-localized. Co-registration of 3D BLI facilitated positioning of bioluminescent signal sources within the tumor, revealing a pattern of multiple clusters of bacteria within tumors.

2   Materials

Prepare all bacterial growth media using de-ionized water and according to the manufacturer's specific instructions. All media should be autoclaved at 121 °C for 15 min prior to use. Adhere to aseptic technique guidelines when handling the biological agents and dispose of the biohazard waste appropriately.

2.1   Bacterial Growth

1. 38 g/l Reinforced clostridial broth (Oxoid).
2. 52.5 g/l Reinforced clostridial agar (Oxoid).
3. 20 g/l LB broth (Sigma).
4. 35 g/l LB agar (Sigma).

5. 0.05 % cysteine-HCl solution in H_2O (1.2 g/20 ml H_2O). Filter sterilize, do not autoclave (Sigma).

6. 10 mg/ml chloramphenicol in EtOH stock solution. Filter sterilize, do not autoclave, store at –20 °C, and add 5 μl per 10 ml of growth media for *B. breve* (Sigma).

7. 100 mg/ml erythromycin in EtOH stock solution. Filter sterilize, do not autoclave, store at –20 °C, and add 30 μl per 10 ml of growth media for *E. coli* (Sigma).

8. Laminar flow hood for aseptic culture of the bacterium.

9. Anaerobic chamber at 37 °C for growth of *B. breve*.

10. Shaking incubator at 37 °C for growth of *E. coli*.

11. Spectrophotometer at 600 nm to measure optical density of the bacterial cultures.

2.2 Tumor Cell Line

1. The HCT116-luc2 cell line (Caliper) was maintained in McCoy's 5a Medium Modified (ATCC) supplemented with 10 % fetal calf serum (FCS), 100 U/ml penicillin, 100 mg/ml streptomycin, and 2 mM L-glutamine and sodium pyruvate.

2. The CT26 murine cell line was maintained in Dulbecco's Modified Eagle's Medium (Sigma) supplemented with 10 % fetal calf serum (FCS).

3. PBS (Sigma).

4. NucleoCounter, for eukaryotic-cell counting (ChemoMetec, Bioimages Ltd).

5. 5 % CO_2 37 °C incubator.

6. Laminar-flow hood for aseptic passaging of the cell line.

2.3 In Vivo Imaging

1. IVIS 100 imaging system or its equivalent is required for 2D imaging and IVIS Spectrum for 3D imaging. Both are capable of in vivo imaging of anesthetized mice (Caliper).

2. D-Luciferin (Caliper).

3. Living Image software for processing of bioluminescence data (Caliper).

4. XGI-8 Gas Anesthesia System (Caliper) with 3 % isoflurane for gas anesthesia of the mice (*see* **Note 1**).

2.4 Animal

1. Mouse model for HCT116-luc2; athymic Crl:NU(NCr)-Fox1nu mice (Charles River).

2. Mouse model for CT26; BALB/c Haplotype: *H-2d* (Harlan, UK).

3. Appropriate animal restrainer and holding facilities (Vet-Tech Solutions, UK).

4. 21 and 28 gauge needles (BD BioSciences).

5. 20 mm pore nylon filter (Falcon, BD BioSciences).

3   Methods

3.1   Tumor Induction

1. For routine tumor induction, the minimum tumorigenic dose of cells (HCT116-luc2 5×10^5; CT26 1×10^6) suspended in 200 µl of serum-free culture medium was injected subcutaneously (s.c.) into the flank of infection-free 6–8-week-old mice using a 21-gauge syringe needle.

2. The viability of cells used for inoculation was greater than 95 % as determined by visual count using a NucleoCounter (*see* **Note 2**).

3. Following tumor establishment, tumors were allowed to grow and develop and were monitored twice weekly (*see* **Note 3**).

4. Tumor volume was calculated according to the formula $V = (ab^2) \Pi/6$, where a is the longest diameter of the tumor and b is the longest diameter perpendicular to the diameter a.

3.2   Bacterial Preparation

1. The bacterial strains used in this protocol were either *E. coli* K-12 MG1655, a nonprotein-toxin-expressing strain, or *B. breve* UCC2003, a commensal probiotic strain, both harboring a luxABCDE cassette that enables the bacteria to be detected by BLI.

2. The bioluminescent derivative of MG1655 was created using the plasmid p16Slux which contains the constitutive P_{HELP}luxABCDE operon [9].

3. The bioluminescent derivative of UCC2003 was created using the plasmid pLuxMC3 [14].

4. *E. coli* MG1655 luxABCDE was grown aerobically at 37 °C in LB medium supplemented with 300 µg/ml erythromycin (Em).

5. *B. breve* UCC2003 containing pLuxMC3 was grown anaerobically (*see* **Note 4**) at 37 °C in MRS medium supplemented with 0.05 % cysteine-HCl and 5 µg/ml chloramphenicol (Cm).

6. For preparation for administration to mice, MG1655 cultures were incubated in LB medium at 37 °C in a shaker at 200 rpm to grow to mid-log phase (optical density at 600 nm). Bacteria were harvested by centrifugation ($6000 \times g$ for 10 min), washed twice with PBS, and diluted in PBS to 1×10^7 colony-forming units (cfu)/ml for iv administration.

7. UCC2003 cultures were initially grown in RCM medium overnight (*see* **Note 5**) and then subcultured at 1 % to MRS medium supplemented with 0.05 % cysteine-HCl. Following a further overnight incubation, the bacteria were harvested by centrifugation ($6000 \times g$ for 10 min), washed twice with PBS containing 0.05 % cysteine-HCl, and diluted in PBS containing 0.05 % cysteine-HCl to 1×10^7 colony-forming units (CFU)/ml for iv administration.

3.3 Bacterial Administration

1. Mice were randomly divided into experimental groups when tumors reached approximately 100 mm³ in volume.

2. For intravenous administration, restrained (*see* **Note 6**) mice each received 10⁶ bacterial cells in 100 μl, injected directly into the lateral tail vein using a 28G syringe needle (*see* **Note 7**).

3. The viable count of each inoculum was determined by retrospective plating onto antibiotic-selective agar.

3.4 2D BLI: Intratumoral Bacteria Imaging

1. 2D in vivo BLI imaging was performed using the IVIS 100.

2. At defined time point post-bacterial administration, mice were anesthetized using the XGI-8 Gas Anesthesia System with 3 % isoflurane (*see* **Note 8**).

3. Whole-body imaging was performed in the IVIS 100 system for 2–5 min at high sensitivity (Fig. 1).

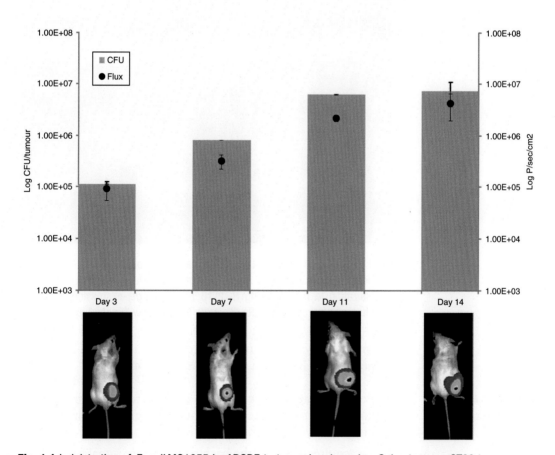

Fig. 1 Administration of *E. coli* MG1655 luxABCDE to tumor-bearing mice. Subcutaneous CT26 tumors were induced in Balb/c mice. *E. coli* MG1655 luxABCDE was administered upon tumor development. Each animal received 10⁶ bacterial cells injected directly into the lateral tail vein. Mice were imaged at four time points during the study (*black dots z-axis* and images) with subsequent recovery of viable bacteria (CFU) from tumors of representative sacrificed mice (*bar graph*). Increase in bacterial number (CFU) and plasmid gene expression specifically in tumors was observed over time (representative mouse illustrated at each time point)

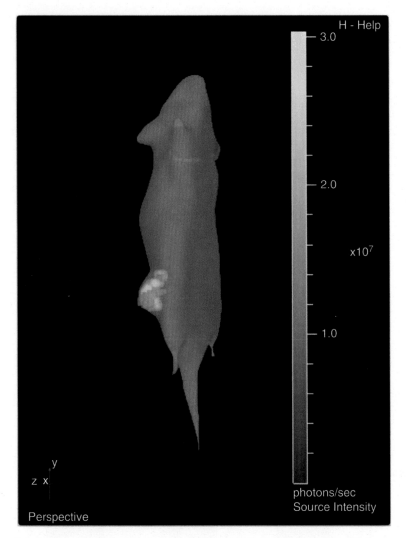

Fig. 2 3D co-localization of tumor and bacterial bioluminescence. 3D tomographic detail of source signal distribution of *B. breve* lux (*green*) 10 days post-iv administration to mice bearing HCT116 *FLuc* (*orange*)-expressing tumors. *B. breve* lux is observed in multiple disparate "clusters" within the tumor

4. Image analysis: regions of interest were identified and quantified using Living Image software (*see* **Note 9**).

3.5 3D BLI:
Intratumoral Bacteria
Imaging

1. For 3D imaging, anesthetized mice were placed in a mouse imaging shuttle inside of the optical imaging system for dorsal imaging (IVIS Spectrum).

2. To acquire images of the bacterial luciferase signal for 3D optical reconstruction, emission filter wavelengths ranging from 500 to 580 nm were used with a bin of 16.

3. Acquisition times of 3–4 min are necessary to maximize the signal to noise ratio (Fig. 2).

4. Image analysis: regions of interest were identified and quantified using Living Image software (*see* **Note 9**).

3.6 3D BLI: Imaging Tumor Fluc and Diffuse Light Imaging Tomography

1. To acquire images of the firefly luciferase emanating from the tumor, luciferin was injected subcutaneously approximately 10 min prior to imaging without moving the animal (Fig. 2).

2. Emission filter wavelengths ranging from 580 to 620 nm were then used with a bin of 8.

3. Acquisition times of 0.5–0.75 min per filter are generally used, depending on the tumor cell line in use.

4. As part of this image acquisition sequence, a structured light image was obtained to define a height map.

5. This map was input for diffuse light imaging tomography (DLIT) reconstruction algorithms for forming a 3D optical image using a non-negative least squares optimization [15].

3.7 Bacterial Recovery from Tumors

1. At four time points post-bacterial administration, the mice were imaged for BLI and then a subset of the animals were euthanized by cervical dislocation.

2. The tumor was aseptically dissected with subsequent recovery of viable bacteria (CFU) from tumors (Fig. 1).

3. To determine the total number of bacteria, the dissected tumors were immediately placed in 5 ml PBS (MG1655) or PBS with 0.05 % cysteine-HCl (UCC2003).

4. Tumors were then homogenized by fine mincing with a scalpel, followed by pushing through a 20 mm pore nylon filter in sterile PBS (supplemented with 0.05 % cysteine-HCl for bifidobacteria).

5. Serial dilutions were plated in triplicate on selective agar; *B. breve* on RCA agar containing 5 μg/ml Cm and *E. coli* on LB agar containing 300 μg/ml Em.

6. Resulting colonies were used to calculate the number of bacterial cells per tissue sample.

7. To confirm that cfu recovered were either *B. breve* containing pLuxMC3 or *E. coli* MG1655luxABCDE, random isolates were spot inoculated onto the appropriate agar either with or without the selective antibiotic and checked by PCR as previously described [9].

8. An increase in bacterial number and plasmid gene expression specifically in tumors was observed over time as illustrated by both BLI and CFU (*see* Fig. 1).

4   Notes

1. Appropriate training on the use of inhalation anesthesia is essential prior to its use.

2. The NucleoCounter can be substituted by a hemocytometer and trypan blue exclusion dye (Gibco).

3. Vernier calipers should be used to monitor tumor growth and development. The same person, ideally, should perform all measurements over time as the technique can be subjective in the early stages of growth.

4. It is essential to maintain a strict anaerobic environment at all times. The most convenient way is to perform all the culturing techniques in an anaerobic hood and then inject the bacteria into the mice immediately following removal from the hood. If this isn't feasible, then a portable anaerobic jar can be used, along with Anaerocult oxygen scavenging sachets, to transport the prepared bacteria in an anaerobic environment until they can be injected to the animals.

5. RCM broth is necessary in order to allow the *B. breve* to grow from frozen stocks. The broth contains low levels of suspended agarose. This broth cannot be used to prepare the bacteria for injection, as centrifuging the culture results in a layer of agarose forming over the cell pellet. Therefore, following an overnight incubation in RCM, the *B. breve* must be subcultured in the more chemically-defined MRS broth which is suitable for centrifugation.

6. Commercial restrainers are available which contain the animal individually and allow the tail to be exposed for injection. The animal should remain in the restrainer for the minimum amount of time possible to avoid distress.

7. Anatomically, there are two lateral tail veins in the mouse tail. Mild heat should be applied using a heat pad under the mouse cage to increase vasodilation prior to injection. A 28G needle, also known as an insulin syringe, is necessary to inject into the tail vein as larger-gauge needles can lead to destruction of the vein. The technique is initially difficult to master and requires an advanced level of competency in animal surgical techniques.

8. Ensure that the animal's nose is securely within the oxygen mask used to deliver the inhalation anesthesia to avoid premature awakening during image acquisition.

9. Regions of interest are always calculated as $p/s/cm^2$.

Acknowledgments

The authors wish to acknowledge Dr. Cormac Gahan and Dr. Susan Joyce for providing lux-tagged *E. coli* MG1655 and relevant funding support from the European Commission Seventh Framework Programme (PIAP- GA-2013-612219-VIP), Science Foundation Ireland/Enterprise Ireland (12/TIDA/B2437), the Irish Health Research Board (HRA_POR/2010/138), and the Irish Cancer Society (CRF11CRO and PCI12TAN).

References

1. Tangney M, Francis KP (2012) In vivo optical imaging in gene & cell therapy. Curr Gene Ther 12:2–11

2. Tangney M, Ahmad S, Collins SA, O'Sullivan GC (2010) Gene therapy for prostate cancer. Postgrad Med 122:166–180

3. Morrissey D, O'Sullivan GC, Tangney M (2010) Tumor targeting with systemically administered bacteria. Curr Gene Ther 10:3–14

4. Collins SA, Guinn BA, Harrison PT, Scallan MF, O'Sullivan GC, Tangney M (2008) Viral vectors in cancer immunotherapy: which vector for which strategy? Curr Gene Ther 8:66–78

5. Baban CK, Cronin M, O'Hanlon D, O'Sullivan GC, Tangney M (2010) Bacteria as vectors for gene therapy of cancer. Bioeng Bugs 1:385–394

6. Yu YA, Zhang Q, Szalay AA (2008) Establishment and characterization of conditions required for tumor colonization by intravenously delivered bacteria. Biotechnol Bioeng 100:567–578

7. Cronin M, Morrissey D, Rajendran S, El Mashad SM, van Sinderen D, O'Sullivan GC et al (2010) Orally administered bifidobacteria as vehicles for delivery of agents to systemic tumors. Mol Ther 18:1397–1407

8. van Pijkeren JP, Morrissey D, Monk IR, Cronin M, Rajendran S, O'Sullivan GC et al (2010) A novel Listeria monocytogenes-based DNA delivery system for cancer gene therapy. Hum Gene Ther 21:405–416

9. Cronin M, Akin AR, Collins SA, Meganck J, Kim JB, Baban CK et al (2012) High resolution in vivo bioluminescent imaging for the study of bacterial tumor targeting. PLoS One 7:e30940

10. Ahmad S, Casey G, Cronin M, Rajendran S, Sweeney P, Tangney M et al (2011) Induction of effective antitumor response after mucosal bacterial vector mediated DNA vaccination with endogenous prostate cancer specific antigen. J Urol 186:687–693

11. Riedel CU, Monk IR, Casey PG, Morrissey D, O'Sullivan GC, Tangney M et al (2007) Improved luciferase tagging system for Listeria monocytogenes allows real-time monitoring in vivo and in vitro. Appl Environ Microbiol 73:3091–3094

12. Baban CK, Cronin M, Akin AR, O'Brien A, Gao X, Tabirca S et al (2012) Bioluminescent bacterial imaging in vivo. J Vis Exp 4:e4318

13. Cheng CM, Lu YL, Chuang KH, Hung WC, Shiea J, Su YC et al (2008) Tumor-targeting prodrug-activating bacteria for cancer therapy. Cancer Gene Ther 15:393–401

14. Cronin M, Sleator RD, Hill C, Fitzgerald GF, van Sinderen D (2008) Development of a luciferase-based reporter system to monitor Bifidobacterium breve UCC2003 persistence in mice. BMC Microbiol 8:161

15. Kuo C, Coquoz O, Troy TL, Xu H, Rice BW (2007) Three-dimensional reconstruction of in vivo bioluminescent sources based on multispectral imaging. J Biomed Opt 12:024007

Chapter 8

Employment of *Salmonella* in Cancer Gene Therapy

Che-Hsin Lee

Abstract

One of the primary limitations of cancer gene therapy is lack of selectivity of the therapeutic gene to tumor cells. Current efforts are focused on discovering and developing tumor-targeting vectors that selectively target only cancer cells but spare normal cells to improve the therapeutic index. The use of preferentially tumor-targeting bacteria as vectors is one of the innovative approaches for the treatment of cancer. This is based on the observation that some obligate or facultative-anaerobic bacteria are capable of multiplying selectively in tumors and inhibiting their growth. In this study, we exploited attenuated *Salmonella* as a tumoricidal agent and a vector to deliver genes for tumor-targeted gene therapy. Attenuated *Salmonella*, carrying a eukaryotic expression plasmid encoding an anti-angiogenic gene, was used to evaluate its' ability for tumor targeting and gene delivery in murine tumor models. We also investigated the use of a polymer to modify or shield *Salmonella* from the pre-existing immune response in the host in order to improve gene delivery to the tumor. These results suggest that tumor-targeted gene therapy using *Salmonella* carrying a therapeutic gene, which exerts tumoricidal and anti-angiogenic activities, represents a promising strategy for the treatment of tumors.

Key words *Salmonella*, Tumor targeting, Gene therapy, Polymer, Antitumor

1 Introduction

The use of bacteria preferentially replicating in tumors as an onco-lytic agent is an innovative approach for cancer treatment. This is based on the observation that some obligate or facultative-anaerobic bacteria are capable of multiplying selectively in tumors and inhibiting their growth [1–4]. Genetically-modified, non-pathogenic bacteria have been tested as potential anti-tumor agents, either to provide direct tumoricidal effects or to deliver tumoricidal molecules. Apart from obligate anaerobes which target hypoxic/necrotic areas of solid tumors, such as *Clostridium* [5] and *Bifidobacterium* [6], *Salmonella* [7], a facultative anaerobe capable of growing under both aerobic and anaerobic conditions, has also been exploited as a potential oncolytic agent [8–10]. In addition, these tumor-targeted bacteria can be used to deliver genes encoding pro-drug-converting enzymes [2], angiogenic

Robert M. Hoffman (ed.), *Bacterial Therapy of Cancer: Methods and Protocols*, Methods in Molecular Biology, vol. 1409,
DOI 10.1007/978-1-4939-3515-4_8, © Springer Science+Business Media New York 2016

inhibitors [11], or cytokines [12], aiming to enhance anti-cancer efficacy.

We examined the capability of *Salmonella* to preferentially accumulate and replicate in tumors as well as to achieve tumor-specific gene delivery [4, 11]. Furthermore, by targeting tumor hypoxia per se and tumor vasculature, we tested the anti-tumor and anti-metastatic effects of *Salmonella*, carrying an anti-angiogenic gene, on a murine tumor model. Our results suggest that by taking advantages of inherent anti-tumor activity and delivery of therapeutic genes to the tumor site, *Salmonella* carrying anti-angiogenic genes has therapeutic potential for the treatment of solid tumors.

In agreement with a clinical study, our previous results indicated that higher anti-*Salmonella* antibody titers in the host resulted in lower amounts of *Salmonella* in the tumor [13]. Anti-*Salmonella* antibodies result in a noticeably lower total number of bacteria in tumor sites and decrease the anti-tumor effect of *Salmonella*. Therefore, the avoidance of neutralizing antibodies has emerged as a key issue in the development of *Salmonella* cancer therapy. We investigated the use of poly(allylamine hydrochloride) (PAH) to modify or shield *Salmonella* from the pre-existing immune response in a host [14]. Because adverse toxic effects caused by bacterial therapy are the main hindrance to clinical development [15], we explored the use of PAH-modified *Salmonella*, which did not induce a large response of inflammatory cytokines; as inflammatory responses would negatively affect the health of the host. PAH also can provide a useful platform for the chemical modification of *Salmonella*, perhaps allowing genes to bind to tumor-targeting *Salmonella*. The combination of tumor-targeting activity of *Salmonella* and the pleiotropic activities of a gene delivery system holds promise for tumor treatment (Fig. 1).

2   Materials

Prepare all solutions using ultrapure water (prepared by purifying de-ionized water to attain a sensitivity of 18 M Ω cm at 25 °C) and analytical grade reagents. Prepare and store all reagents at room temperature.

Luria broth (LB) (*see* **Note 1**).

LB agar (*see* **Note 2**).

Glycerol (*see* **Note 3**).

50 mg poly(allylamine hydrochloride) (PAH; MW: 15,000; Sigma-Aldrich) (*see* **Note 4**).

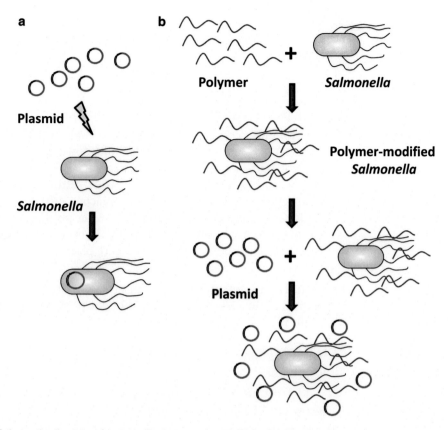

Fig. 1 Schematic diagram of two methods to construct *Salmonella* carrying a gene for tumor therapy. (**a**) Transformation of plasmid DNA into *Salmonella* by electroporation. (**b**) *Salmonella* carrying plasmid DNA using layer-by-layer technology

3   Methods

3.1   *Salmonella* Transformed with a Therapeutic Gene by Electroporation

1. Add a colony of *Salmonella* to a 25 mL LB flask; grow overnight.

2. Add 1 mL from the overnight culture to a 250 mL LB flask; grow until bacteria are in log phase.

3. Divide the culture into two centrifuge flasks.

4. Centrifuge at $2600 \times g$ for 15 min in a 4 °C centrifuge.

5. Discard the supernatants and resuspend the cell pellets in 2×125 mL 10 % glycerol.

6. Suspend pelleted cells in 1 mL 10 % glycerol; combine fractions and split into 100 μL aliquots.

7. Place 1–2 μL (1 μg/μL) of plasmid in the bottom of a labeled Eppendorf tube. Add 20 μL of just-thawed *Salmonella*.

8. Open the electroporation chamber and pipet 20 µL of the bacteria-plasmid mixture, suspended between the electrodes of the chamber.

9. Check settings or set to pulse control = 330 µF, low omega, and fast-charge rate.

10. Turn power switches on for both power boosters.

11. Charge pulse control by setting the CHARGE/ARM switch to CHARGE and then press and hold down the UP voltage control button until the voltage reading is ~410 V. Release button and quickly switch to the ARM setting. The voltage will begin to fall slowly. When it reaches 400 V, press the TRIGGER button and hold for 1 s. After pulsing, verify that the pulse control unit indicates <20 V. Remove suspended cells from the chambers with a pipet and place in 1 mL LB to recover for 1 h. at 37 °C in a shaker.

12. Plate 100 µL on appropriate plates (with antibiotic that corresponds to the resistance conferred by the plasmid). Grow overnight in a 37 °C incubator.

3.2 Preparation of DNA-PAH-Modified Salmonella

1. Add a colony of *Salmonella* to a 25 mL LB flask; grow overnight.

2. Add 1 mL from the overnight culture to a 250 mL LB flask; grow until bacteria are in log phase.

3. Divide the culture into two centrifuge flasks.

4. Centrifuge at $2600 \times g$ for 15 min in a 4 °C centrifuge.

5. Discard the supernatants and resuspend the cell pellets in 2×125 mL 10 % glycerol.

6. Suspend the pelleted cells in 1 mL 10 % glycerol; combine fractions and split into 100 µL aliquots.

7. Place 1 mL (5 mg/mL) PAH in an Eppendorf tube. Add 100 µL just-thawed *Salmonella*.

8. Incubate on a shaker for 15 min (37 °C) and then centrifuge (10 min at $1000 \times g$).

9. Discard the excess PAH solution and disperse the *Salmonella* and wash three times in water.

10. Place 1 mL (5 µg) of plasmid in an Eppendorf tube. Add 100 µL PAH-modified *Salmonella*.

11. Incubate on a shaker for 15 min (37 °C) and then centrifuge (10 min at $1000 \times g$).

12. Discard the excess PAH solution and disperse the *Salmonella* and wash three times in water.

4 Notes

1. Luria broth (LB): trypton 10 g, yeast extract 5 g, and sodium chloride 5 g. Add water to a volume of 1000 mL. Autoclave at 121 °C for at least 15 min. Store at 4 °C.

2. LB agar: bacterial agar 15 g. Add LB to a volume of 1000 mL. Autoclave at 121 °C for at least 15 min. Store at 4 °C.

3. Glycerol: autoclave at 121 °C for at least 15 min, store at 4 °C.

4. 50 mg poly(allylamine hydrochloride) (PAH; MW: 15,000; Sigma-Aldrich): add water to a volume of 10 mL. The solution is purified by drawing it up a syringe through a filter.

References

1. Pawelek JM, Low KB, Bermudes D (2003) Bacteria as tumour-targeting vectors. Lancet Oncol 4:548–556

2. Pawelek JM, Low KB, Bermudes D (1997) Tumor-targeted *Salmonella* as a novel anticancer vector. Cancer Res 57:4537–4544

3. Zhao M, Yang M, Li XM, Jiang P, Baranov E, Li S, Xu M, Penman S, Hoffman RM (2005) Tumor-targeting bacterial therapy with amino acid auxotrophs of GFP-expressing *Salmonella typhimurium*. Proc Natl Acad Sci U S A 102:755–760

4. Lee CH, Wu CL, Shiau AL (2004) Endostatin gene therapy delivered by *Salmonella choleraesuis* in murine tumor models. J Gene Med 6:1382–1393

5. Dang LH, Bettegowda C, Huso DL, Kinzler KW, Vogelstein B (2001) Combination bacteriolytic therapy for the treatment of experimental tumors. Proc Natl Acad Sci U S A 98:15155–15160

6. Yazawa K, Fujimori M, Amano J, Kano Y, Taniguchi S (2000) *Bifidobacterium longum* as a delivery system for cancer gene therapy: selective localization and growth in hypoxic tumors. Cancer Gene Ther 7:269–274

7. Lee CH, Wu CL, Tai YS, Shiau AL (2005) Systemic administration of attenuated *Salmonella choleraesuis* in combination with cisplatin for cancer therapy. Mol Ther 11:707–716

8. Lee CH, Hsieh JL, Wu CL, Hsu PY, Shiau AL (2011) T cell augments the antitumor activity of tumor-targeting *Salmonella*. Appl Microbiol Biotechnol 90:1381–1388

9. Liu F, Zhang L, Hoffman RM, Zhao M (2010) Vessel destruction by tumor-targeting *Salmonella typhimurium* A1-R is enhanced by high tumor vascularity. Cell Cycle 9:4518–4524

10. Nagakura C, Hayashi K, Zhao M, Yamauchi K, Yamamoto N, Tsuchiya H, Tomita K, Bouvet M, Hoffman RM (2009) Efficacy of a genetically-modified *Salmonella typhimurium* in an orthotopic human pancreatic cancer in nude mice. Anticancer Res 29:1873–1878

11. Lee CH, Wu CL, Shiau AL (2005) Systemic administration of attenuated *Salmonella choleraesuis* carrying thrombospondin-1 gene leads to tumor-specific transgene expression, delayed tumor growth and prolonged survival in the murine melanoma model. Cancer Gene Ther 12:175–182

12. Ganai S, Arenas RB, Forbes NS (2009) Tumour-targeted delivery of TRAIL using *Salmonella typhimurium* enhances breast cancer survival in mice. Br J Cancer 101:1683–1691

13. Lee CH, Wu CL, Chen SH, Shiau AL (2009) Humoral immune responses inhibit the antitumor activities mediated by *Salmonella enterica* serovar Choleraesuis. J Immunother 32:376–388

14. Lee CH, Lin YH, Hsieh JL, Chen MC, Kuo WL (2013) A polymer coating applied to *Salmonella* prevents the binding of *Salmonella*-specific antibodies. Int J Cancer 132:717–725

15. Lee CH (2012) Engineering bacteria toward tumor targeting for cancer treatment: current state and perspectives. Appl Microbiol Biotechnol 93:517–523

Chapter 9

Development of a Targeted Gene-Delivery System Using *Escherichia coli*

Chung-Jen Chiang, Chih-Hsiang Chang, Yun-Peng Chao, and Ming-Ching Kao

Abstract

A gene-delivery system based on microbes is useful for development of targeted gene therapy of non-phagocytic cancer cells. Here, the feasibility of the delivery system is illustrated by targeted delivery of a transgene (i.e., eukaryotic GFP) by *Escherichia coli* to HER2/*neu*-positive cancer cells. An *E. coli* strain was engineered with surface display of the anti-HER2/*neu* affibody. To release the gene cargo, a programmed lysis system based on phage φX174 gene E was introduced into the *E. coli* strain. As a result, 3 % of HER2/*neu*-positive cells that were infected with engineered *E. coli* were able to express the GFP.

Key words Bacterial carrier, Targeted delivery, HER2/*neu*, Bactofection

1 Introduction

Vehicles based on bacteria have been developed to deliver transgenics to mammalian cells, a process known as bactofection [1]. The bacterial delivery system is a nonviral vector and considered as a safe method for gene therapy [2]. One promising approach with the bacterial vectors is to deliver therapeutic cargos to tumors. This requires that bacterial vectors have the ability to selectively recognize and invade tumors. After internalization, the gene cargos carried by bacterial vectors are freely released. However, many challenges are present in the bactofection process.

The first limiting step in bactofection is the selective entry of the bacterial vector into cancer cells [1]. To address this issue, the anti-HER2/*neu* affibody (ZH2) was displayed on *E. coli* surface via the anchoring motif Lpp-OmpA. The anchoring motif contains the Lpp region that directs the passenger motif across the inner membrane of *E. coli*. Meanwhile, the OmpA domain helps anchor the passenger on the outer membrane [3]. Consequently, *E. coli* with surface display of ZH2 enables selective invasion of

Robert M. Hoffman (ed.), *Bacterial Therapy of Cancer: Methods and Protocols*, Methods in Molecular Biology, vol. 1409,
DOI 10.1007/978-1-4939-3515-4_9, © Springer Science+Business Media New York 2016

HER2/*neu*-positive cells, with the invasion efficiency reaching 30 % [4].

The free release of transgenic cargos carried by bacterial vectors appears to be the second limiting step in bactofection [1]. Therefore, the phage φX174 gene E, under thermal regulation, was transfected into *E. coli*. This phage gene encodes a lysin gene that causes the formation of a trans-membrane tunnel across the inner and outer membrane of *E. coli* [5]. Consequently, approximately 3 % of HER2/*neu*-positive cells that were infected with the engineered *E. coli* carrying CMV-promoter-driven GFP were shown to exhibit green fluorescence 24 h after bactofection [4].

2   Materials

Prepare all solutions using ultrapure water (prepare by purifying de-ionized water to attain a sensitivity of 18 MΩ cm at 25 °C) and analytical-grade reagents. Prepare and store all reagents at room temperature (unless indicated otherwise). Follow all regulations when disposing waste materials.

2.1   Bacterial Strains

BL21-GFP (*see* **Note 1**).

BL21-GFP/pET-Her2M (*see* **Note 2**).

BL21(DE3)/pBAD-LoAZH2 (*see* **Note 3**).

BL21-GFP/pBAD-LoAZH2 (*see* **Note 4**).

BL21(DE3)/pBAD-LoAZH2/pCL-φXE2-hlyA (*see* **Note 5**).

BL21-GFP/pBAD-LoAZH2/pCL-φXE2-hlyA (*see* **Note 6**).

BL21(DE3)/pBAD-LoAZH2/pCL-φXE2-hlyA/pBac-EGFP (*see* **Note 7**).

2.2   Cell Lines (See Note 8)

Human Breast Cancer Cell Lines

MDA-MB-231 (ATCC number: HTB-26).

SKBR-3 (ATCC number: HTB-30).

2.3   Materials

Mouse anti-6xHis monoclonal antibody (Genemark Technology Co. Ltd, Taiwan).

TRITC-conjugated anti-mouse IgG (Jackson Immuno Research, West Grove, PA, USA).

Phalloidin-TRITC (Sigma-Aldrich, St. Louis, MO, USA).

DAPI (Sigma-Aldrich).

9G6 anti-HER2/*neu* primary antibody (Santa Cruz Biotechnol., Dallas, TX, USA).

Trypsin-EDTA (HyClone Lab. Inc., Logan, UT, USA).

2.4 Equipment	Fluorescence microscopy (Olympus IX71, Tokyo, Japan).
	BD FACSCanto (BD Bioscience, Franklin Lakes, NJ, USA).
	Diva software (De novo Software, Los Angeles, CA, USA).
	FlowJo (TreeStar, Ashland, OR, USA).
	Confocal microscopy (Leica, LCS SP2, Wetzlar, Germany).
	LAS AF (Leica)

3 Methods

3.1 Plasmid
Construction

3.1.1 Plasmid
pφT7-GFPuv

1. Create this plasmid by ligation of a DNA fragment, removed from plasmid pET28-GFPuv by *Sac*I-*Sph*I digestion, into plasmid pPhi80-Tc [6]. This plasmid carries a DNA cassette consisting of T7 promoter-driven GFP.

3.1.2 Plasmid
pET-Her2M

1. Amplify the anti-HER2/*neu* ML39 ScFv from plasmid pACgp67B-Her2mP (Addgene Inc.) using the polymerase chain reaction (PCR) with primer YC1101 and YC1102.

2. Digest the ML39 ScFv-containing DNA with *Nco*I-*Eco*RI and ligate into plasmid pET-20b (Novagene Co.) to obtain plasmid pET-Her2.

3. Obtain the *misL* gene of *Salmonella typhimurium* LT2 by PCR with primer YC1103 and YC1104. After *Eco*RI-*Hind*III cleavage, incorporate the resulting DNA into plasmid pET-Her2 to produce plasmid pET-Her2M [5].

3.1.3 Plasmid
pBAD-LoAZH2

1. Synthesize the ZH2 DNA motif and confirm with DNA sequencing by Mission Biotech. Co. (Taiwan). It contains two identical domains of $Z_{HER2:342}$ [7] separated by a linker.

2. Incorporate the synthesized DNA into plasmid pLOA [8] to result in plasmid pLOA-ZH.

3. Subsequently, recover the DNA from plasmid pLOA-ZH by *Hind*III-*Xba*I cleavage and splice into plasmid pBAD33 [9] to give plasmid pBAD-LoAZH2 [4].

3.1.4 Plasmid
pCL-φXE2-hlyA

1. To reduce the basal expression level at 37 °C, mutate λ P_{RM} and the P_R promoter of plasmid pPL452 [10] according to a previous report [11]. Carry out by site-directed mutagenesis [12] to give plasmid pPL452M with two pairs of primers, YC1105/YC1106 and YC1107/YC1108.

2. From phage φX174 DNA, amplify gene E by PCR with primers YC1109 and YC1110.

3. Pre-treat the PCR DNA with *Eco*RI-*Nde*I and ligate into plasmid pPL452M to produce pPL-φXE.

4. Synthesize the *hlyA* gene of *L. monocytogenes* by PCR from plasmid pGB2Ω-inv-hly [13], using primers YC1111 and YC1112.

5. Digest with *Xho*I-*Sma*I, and incorporate the PCR DNA into plasmid pPL-ϕXE to give plasmid pPL-ϕXE-hlyA.

6. Recover the DNA containing ϕX174 gene E and *hlyA* from plasmid pPL-ϕXE-hlyA by *Pst*I-*Nru*I cleavage.

7. Splice the recovered DNA into plasmid pCL1920 to give plasmid pCL-ϕXE2-hlyA [4].

3.2 Analysis of the Bacterial Surface by Immunostaining and Flow Cytometry

1. Grow bacteria and induce by adding l-arabinose.

2. After induction for 4 h, harvest bacteria, wash, and resuspend in phosphate buffer (pH 7.4).

3. Withdraw bacteria (1×10^9) and treat with 500 µL 0.25 % trypsin-EDTA at 37 °C for 2 min.

4. Terminate the digestion with 500 µL 10 % FBS/DMEM-F12 medium on ice.

5. Fix the uninduced, induced, and trypsinized bacteria in 3.7 % paraformaldehyde for 30 min.

6. Wash the BSA-blocked bacterial cells three times with PBS and incubate with 1:200 diluted mouse anti-6xHis monoclonal antibody at room temperature for 1 h.

7. Rinse the bacteria and expose to a 200-fold dilution of FITC-conjugated anti-mouse IgG for 1 h.

8. After washing with PBS, mount bacterial cells on glass slides for analysis by fluorescence microscopy.

9. Use 10,000 bacteria for measurement of green fluorescence with a BD FACSCanto. Further analyze data with a Diva software and FlowJo.

3.3 Infection of Tumor Cells with Bacteria

Seed human tumor cells into 12- and 24-well plates with cover slips for flow cytometry and microscopy, respectively.

1. Wash the harvested bacteria twice with serum-free medium, dilute in the serum-free medium, and then add to each well to achieve the required multiplicity of infection (MOI).

2. Incubate in a humidified atmosphere of 5 % CO_2 at 37 °C for 3 h.

3. Wash the culture plates three times with PBS to remove unbound bacteria (*see* **Note 11**) and then incubate at 42 °C for 60 min for thermal induction (*see* **Note 12**).

4. Apply 50 µg/mL gentamicin for 1 h at 37 °C to eliminate un-internalized bacteria.

5. Incubate the treated cells in a humidified CO_2 incubator at 37 °C until observation (Fig. 1, lower panel).

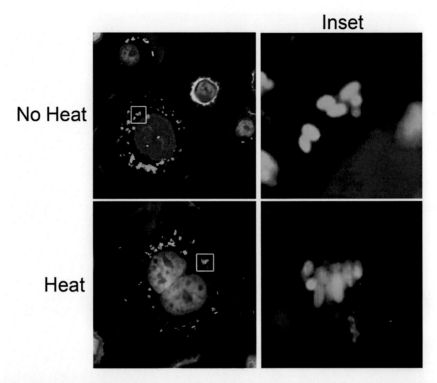

Fig. 1 Analysis of invasion of ZH2-presenting *E. coli* and heat-induced autolysis, by fluorescence microscopy. For clear visualization by fluorescence microscopy, the cell nucleus (*blue*) and cytoskeleton (*red*) were stained by DAPI and phalloidin, respectively. After infection with BL21-GFP/pBAD-LoAZH2/pCL-φXE2-hlyA strain, fluorescence images of SKBR-3 cells were acquired in the *green*, *red*, and *blue* channels and merged. (*Upper*) The invading bacteria were observed by green fluorescence. The magnified image of the inset. (*Lower*) After heat-induced bacterial autolysis, the *green* fluorescence was disappeared is shown in the *right* panel

3.4 Assessment of Bacterial Invasion Efficiency

1. After infection with bacteria for 3 h, wash cancer cells with PBS twice, collect, and then treat with 0.2 % EDTA/PBS.

2. Wash the harvested cells twice with PBS and then fix in 1 % paraformaldehyde.

3. The percentage of 10,000 cells that emit bacteria-producing GFP is determined with a BD FACSCanto. Further analyze data with Diva software and FlowJo.

3.5 Analysis of Bacterial Internalization by Fluorescence and Confocal Microscopy

1. After bacterial infection, wash cells with PBS and fix in 3.7 % paraformaldehyde for 30 min at room temperature.

2. Wash cells three times with PBS and subsequently block with 3 % BSA in PBS. If observe by fluorescence microscopy, go to **step 3**; if by confocal microscopy, go to **step 5**.

3. For fluorescence microscopy, stain cells with 5 μg/mL phalloidin-TRITC and 1 μg/mL DAPI.

4. Mount cells, washed with PBS, on glass slides for observation by fluorescence microscopy (Fig. 1, upper panel).

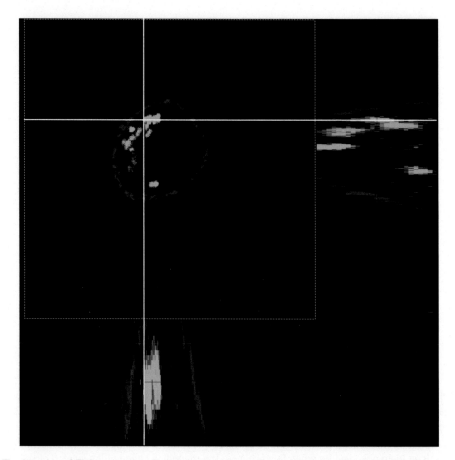

Fig. 2 The invasion of ZH2-presenting *E. coli* observed by confocal microscopy. For further analysis by confocal microscopy, immunostaining of the infected cells was conducted by incubation with anti-HER2/*neu* primary antibody, followed by application of TRITC-conjugated anti-mouse IgG (*red*). Furthermore, two three-dimensional reconstruction sections are shown below (X–Z section) and to the *right* (Y–Z section) of the merge panel. The images demonstrate the appearance of the internalized bacteria (*green*) in the cytoplasm surrounded by HER2/*neu* receptors (*red*)

5. For confocal microscopy, stain cells with 9G6 anti-HER2/*neu* primary antibody for 1 h at room temperature.

6. After washing three times with PBS, add TRITC-conjugated anti-mouse IgG to cells for 1 h.

7. Wash stained cells with PBS and mount on glass slides for analysis by confocal microscopy. For each sample, take a composite image of 20 sections with a 0.8 μm shift in the z-axis and combine with LAS AF (Fig. 2).

3.6 Assessment of Internalized Bacteria in Tumor Cells

1. Assay the average number of bacteria that invade one cell at an MOI of 200:1.

2. After infection, wash tumor cells with PBS.

3. Lyse in 0.2 % Triton X-100 at 37 °C for 10 min.

4. Plate serial dilutions of the cell lysate on LB agars. Incubate at 37 °C overnight and then count the bacterial colony forming units (CFC).

3.7 Analysis of GFP Expression in Tumor Cells by Flow Cytometry

1. Incubate cancer cells with bacteria for 3 h.

2. Collect the cells and fix in 1 % paraformaldehyde at 0, 24, 48, and 72 h.

3. Quantify the number of cells emitting fluorescence with a BD FACSCanto.

4. Further analyze the data with Diva software and FlowJo.

5. Perform the experiment in triplicate and assay 20,000 cells each time.

4 Notes

1. This bacterial strain is generated by integrating plasmid pφT7-GFPuv (*see* Subheading 3.1.1) into the genome of strain BL21(DE3) as previously described [6].

2. Purify plasmid pET-Her2M (*see* Subheading 3.1.2) and transform it into BL21-GFP using a chemical method. The transformant is selected on a LB agar plate, supplemented with 50 μg/mL ampicillin. A single colony is picked and cultured in LB medium [14], supplemented with 50 μg/mL ampicillin, at 37 °C overnight and re-inoculated at a turbidity of 0.08 to grow to 0.3 at 550 nm (OD_{550}) at which time 50 μM IPTG is added to induce protein production for 4 h. Bacteria are harvested by centrifugation, washed, and resuspended in phosphate buffer (pH 7.4).

3. Purify plasmid pBAD-LoAZH2 (*see* Subheading 3.1.3) and transform it into BL21(DE3) using a chemical method. The transformant is selected in LB agar supplemented with 20 μg/mL chloramphenicol. A single colony is picked and cultured in LB medium supplemented with 20 μg/mL chloramphenicol at 37 °C overnight and re-inoculated at a turbidity of 0.08 to grow to 0.3 at 550 nm at which time 50 μMl-arabinose is added to induce protein production for 4 h. Bacteria are harvested by centrifugation, washed, and resuspended in phosphate buffer (pH 7.4).

4. Purify plasmid pBAD-LoAZH2 (*see* Subheading 3.1.3) and transform into BL21-GFP (*see* **Note 1**) using a chemical method. The transformant is selected in LB agar supplemented with 20 μg/mL chloramphenicol. A single colony is picked and cultured in LB medium supplemented with 20 μg/mL chloramphenicol at 37 °C overnight and re-inoculated at a turbidity of 0.08 to grow to 0.3 at 550 nm at which time 50 μMl-arabinose and 50 μM IPTG are added to induce protein production for 4 h. Bacteria are harvested by centrifugation, washed, and resuspended in phosphate buffer (pH 7.4).

5. Purify plasmid pCL-φXE2-hlyA (*see* Subheading 3.1.4) and transform into BL21(DE3)/pBAD-LoAZH2 (*see* **Note 3**) using a chemical method. The transformant is selected on a LB agar plate supplemented with 20 μg/mL chloramphenicol and 10 μg/mL streptomycin (*see* **Notes 9** and **10**). A single colony is picked and cultured in LB medium supplemented with 20 μg/mL chloramphenicol and 10 μg/mL streptomycin, at 30 °C overnight and re-inoculated to grow from turbidity of 0.08–0.3 at 550 nm at 37 °C. Upon reaching a turbidity of 0.3 at OD_{550}, 50 μM l-arabinose is added to induce protein production for 4 h. Bacteria are harvested by centrifugation, washed, and resuspended in phosphate buffer (pH 7.4).

6. Purify plasmid pCL-φXE2-hlyA (*see* Subheading 3.1.4) and transform it into BL21-GFP/pBAD-LoAZH2 (*see* **Note 4**) using a chemical method. The transformant is selected on a LB agar plate supplemented with 20 μg/mL chloramphenicol and 10 μg/mL streptomycin (*see* **Notes 9** and **10**). A single colony is picked and cultured in LB medium supplemented with 20 μg/mL chloramphenicol and 10 μg/mL streptomycin at 30 °C overnight and re-inoculated to grow from turbidity of 0.08–0.3 at 550 nm at 37 °C. Upon reaching a turbidity 0.3 at OD_{550}, 50 μM l-arabinose and 50 μM IPTG are added to induce protein production for 4 h. Bacteria are harvested by centrifugation, washed, and resuspended in phosphate buffer (pH 7.4).

7. Purify plasmid pBac-EGFP and transform into BL21(DE3)/ pBAD-LoAZH2/ pCL-φXE2-hlyA (*see* **Note 5**) using a chemical method. The transformant is selected on a LB agar plate supplemented with 20 μg/mL chloramphenicol, 10 μg/mL streptomycin, and 50 μg/mL kanamycin (*see* **Notes 9** and **10**). A single colony is picked and cultured in LB medium supplemented with 20 μg/mL chloramphenicol, 10 μg/mL streptomycin, and 50 μg/mL kanamycin at 30 °C overnight and re-inoculated from turbidity of 0.08–0.3 at 550 nm (OD_{550}) at 37 °C at which time 50 μM l-arabinose is added to induce protein production for 4 h. Bacteria are harvested by centrifugation, washed, and resuspended in phosphate buffer (pH 7.4).

8. Cell lines are cultured in DEME/F12 medium (HyClone Lab. Inc., USA) supplemented with 10 % fetal bovine serum (FBS) and cultured at 37 °C in a humidified atmosphere of 5 % CO_2 with an initial confluence of 20 %. The medium is changed every 2 days. The day before experiments, cells are detached with 0.25 % trypsin-EDTA (HyClone Lab. Inc., USA) at 37 °C for 2 min and collected by centrifugation. Collected cells are washed with PBS and counted with a hemocytometer. Cells are resuspended and seeded into a 24-well plate (1×10^5 cells per well) and 12-well plate (2×10^5 cells per well) in DEME/ F12 medium supplemented with 10 % FBS.

9. The growth rate of pCL-φXE2-hlyA transformants was slow and needed much time.

10. If the multiple transformation of pCL-φXE2-hlyA failed, try to transform pCL-φXE2-hlyA first before any other plasmid.

11. The washes after bactofection are critical for prevention of growth of bacteria in the cell culture medium.

12. Longer heat induction after bactofection was inefficient in improving bacterial lysis.

Acknowledgments

This work is supported by Feng Chia University (08G27501), National Science Council of Taiwan (NSC101-2221-E-035-0575-MY3, NSC102-2622-E-035- 005-CC1), and China Medical University (CMU98-C-11).

References

1. Palffy R, Gardlik R, Hodosy J, Behuliak M, Resko P, Radvansky J, Celec P (2006) Bacteria in gene therapy: bactofection versus alternative gene therapy. Gene Ther 13:101–105

2. Vassaux G, Nitcheu J, Jezzard S, Lemoine NR (2006) Bacterial gene therapy strategies. J Pathol 208:290–298

3. Lee SY, Choi JH, Xu Z (2003) Microbial cell-surface display. Trends Biotechnol 21:45–52

4. Chang CH, Cheng WJ, Kao MC, Chiang CJ, Chao YP (2011) Engineering of *Escherichia coli* for targeted delivery of transgenes to HER2/*neu*-positive tumor cells. Biotechnol Bioeng 108:1662–1672

5. Paukner S, Stiedl T, Kudela P, Bizik J, Laham FA, Lubitz W (2006) Bacterial ghosts as a novel advanced targeting system for drug and DNA delivery. Expert Opin Drug Deliv 3:11–22

6. Chiang CJ, Chen PT, Chao YP (2008) Replicon-free and markerless methods for genomic insertion of DNAs in phage attachment sites and controlled expression of chromosomal genes in *Escherichia coli*. Biotechnol Bioeng 101:985–995

7. Orlova A, Magnusson M, Eriksson TLJ, Nilsson M, Larsson B, Hoiden-Guthenberg I, Widstrom C, Carlsson J, Tolmachev V, Stahl S et al (2006) Tumor imaging using a picomolar affinity HER2 binding affibody molecule. Cancer Res 66:4339–4348

8. Wang JY, Chao YP (2006) Immobilization of cells with surface-displayed chitin-binding domain. Appl Environ Microbiol 72:927–931

9. Guzman LM, Belin D, Carson MJ, Beckwith J (1995) Tight regulation, modulation, and high-level expression by vectors containing the arabinose P_{BAD} promoter. J Bacteriol 177:4121–4130

10. Christopher AL, Penelope EL, Dixon NE (1996) Stable high-copy-number bacteriophage λ promoter vectors for overproduction of proteins in Escherichia coli. Gene 176:49–53

11. Jechlinger W, Glocker J, Haidinger W, Matis A, Szostak MP, Lubitz W (2005) Modulation of gene expression by promoter mutants of the λ *cI*857/P_{RM}/P_R system. J Biotechnol 116:11–20

12. Chiang CJ, Chern JT, Wang JY, Chao YP (2008) Facile immobilization of evolved *Agrobacterium radiobacter* carbamoylase with high thermal and oxidative stability. J Agric Food Chem 56:6348–6354

13. Grillot-Courvalin C, Goussard S, Huetz F, Ojcius DM, Courvalin P (1998) Functional gene transfer from intracellular bacteria to mammalian cells. Nat Biotechnol 16:862–866

14. Miller JH (1972) Experiments in molecular genetics. Cold Spring Harbor Laboratory, Cold Spring Harbor, New York

Chapter 10

Isolation and Analysis of Suppressor Mutations in Tumor-Targeted *msbB Salmonella*

K. Brooks Low, Sean R. Murray, John Pawelek, and David Bermudes

Abstract

Tumor-targeted *Salmonella* offers a promising approach to the delivery of therapeutics for the treatment of cancer. The *Salmonella* strains used, however, must be stably attenuated in order to provide sufficient safety for administration. Approaches to the generation of attenuated *Salmonella* strains have included deletion of the *msbB* gene that is responsible for addition of the terminal myristol group to lipid A. In the absence of myristoylation, lipid A is no longer capable of inducing septic shock, resulting in a significant enhancement in safety. However, *msbB Salmonella* strains also exhibit an unusual set of additional physiological characteristics, including sensitivities to NaCl, EGTA, deoxycholate, polymyxin, and CO_2. Suppressor mutations that compensate for these sensitivities include *somA*, *Suwwan*, *pmrA^C*, and *zwf*. We describe here methods for isolation of strains with compensatory mutations that suppress these types of sensitivities and techniques for determining their underlying genetic changes and analysis of their effects in murine tumor models.

Key words *Salmonella*, Tumor-targeting, Antitumor efficacy, *msbB*, Myristoylation, Lipid A, *somA*, Suwwan, *pmrA^C*, *zwf*, Suppressor analysis, Epistasis, Pseudo-reversion, Tolerance acquisition, Compensatory mutations, Rescue mutations, Chemical conditionality

1 Introduction

There is a long history of clinical observations connecting the co-occurrence of bacterial infections with spontaneous cancer remissions in humans [1]. Among the early investigators trying to exploit those observations and use artificially-initiated bacterial infections to induce anticancer therapeutic effects was William B. Coley [2]. Coley's original studies [3] which used the live gram-positive bacterium now termed Group A *Streptococcus* or *S. pyogenes* were inspired by the work of Fehleisen [4]. Coley subsequently experimented with mixed bacterial extracts from *S. pyogenes* and *Serratia marcesans* that also produced anti-tumor effects and were safer than live bacteria [2]. The later work by Coley is widely regarded as having been the forerunner to modern immuno-therapeutics [1].

Robert M. Hoffman (ed.), *Bacterial Therapy of Cancer: Methods and Protocols*, Methods in Molecular Biology, vol. 1409, DOI 10.1007/978-1-4939-3515-4_10, © Springer Science+Business Media New York 2016

Other early uses of live bacteria for the treatment of cancer were conducted with anaerobic bacteria of the genus *Clostridium* [5–7]. Because solid tumors have an irregular blood supply, they are hypoxic and therefore conducive to germination of anaerobic spores and the growth of the bacteria within the tumor [8, 9]. Recent investigations of live bacteria for the treatment of tumors, which include studies using the genera *Bifidobacterium*, *Clostridium*, *Escherichia*, *Listeria*, and *Salmonella*, represent an area of rapidly-growing interest because of their potential to lead to novel cancer therapeutics [10, 11].

Salmonella sp. are unique among the different bacterial genera that are being explored as anti-cancer therapeutics [10, 11]. *Salmonella* have evolved a dynamic ability to interact with a variety of cell types including epithelial cells and macrophages, co-opting signal-transduction pathways to enter into non-phagocytic cells and to overcome elimination by the innate immune system as well as targeting immuno-privileged sites such as tumors which contributes to their anti-cancer properties [12–17]. *Salmonella* are highly tractable from a genetic standpoint, and are amenable to a variety of genetic manipulations that allow strains with different properties to be rapidly generated and tested for desirable features, including achieving safety, while maintaining anti-tumor activity. Although human clinical studies are currently being conducted on the gram-positive bacteria *Listeria* and *Clostridium* [18–20], at the present time, *Salmonella* are the only gram-negative bacteria to have been shown to be safe by intravenous administration in an FDA-sanctioned human clinical trial [21–23]. Safety in those bacteria was primarily achieved by deletion of the *msbB* gene, which both dramatically reduced the virulence of the strain and the ability of its lipid-A endotoxin to elicit TNFα and induce septic shock [15, 21]. However, it is important to note that other tumor-targeting *Salmonella typhimurium* such as the strain A1-R, that is not an *msbB* mutant, may not require suppressor mutations [24–27]. Also, there is a current clinical trial of a non-*msbB* orally-administered *Salmonella typhimurium* expressing IL2 [28].

In *Salmonella*, *msbB* mutants exhibit an unusual set of physiological sensitivities that we have previously investigated. Surprisingly, the mutations that we isolated that compensate for these sensitivities are mostly null (deletion) mutations in structural genes that result in restoration of growth phenotypes (Table 1).

1.1 Suppressor Mutations

In our studies describing the deletion of *msbB* in *Salmonella* that eliminated TNFα-mediated septic shock [15, 29], we originally noted that we had used a faster growing derivative of the strain that grew somewhat better on conventional Luria-Bertani (LB) medium. We subsequently studied that and several other spontaneous derivatives and found that they exhibited a number of alterations from the parent strain [30]. These novel sensitivities included

Table 1
***Salmonella* suppressor mutations of *msbB*[a]-induced sensitivities**

Phenotype	Genotype	Type of mutation	Effect on growth phenotype	Reference
NaCl resistance in conventional LB media	*somA (ybjX)*	Null	+	[30]
EGTA resistance in LB-no-salt media	*somA (ybjX)*	Null	+	[30]
Bile salts resistance in MacConkey media	*ΔSuwwan*[b]	Null[b]	+	[31]
EGTA and NaCl resistance in LB-no-salt media	*ΔSuwwan*[b]	Null[b]	+	[31]
Polymyxin and EGTA resistance	*pmrA(con)*	Constitutive	+	[32]
CO_2 resistance	*Zwf*	Null	+	[33]

[a]*msbB* (multicopy suppressor of *htrB*, the second one of two designated "*B*"; [34], also known as also known as *mlt* [35], *waaN* [36], and *lpxM* [37]
[b]Suwwan is a large, approximately 100 Kb, deletion that results from recombination of two IS*200* elements [31]

physiological salt concentrations, chelators such as EDTA, MacConkey media (which contains bile salts including deoxycholate [30, 31]), polymyxin [32] and CO_2 [33].

"*Suppressor mutations*," in contrast to "*suppressor genes*" that code for functional elements (such as p53) that play a role in preventing the development of cancer [38], are secondary mutations that counteract, compensate or revert the phenotypic effects of an existing primary mutation. They can be either intra-genic ("*intra-genic suppressors*"), occurring within the same gene or locus as the primary mutation, or extra-genic ("*extragenic suppressors*"), occurring outside the same gene or locus as the primary mutation. Research on suppressor mutations has had a far-reaching impact on molecular genetics, from the early studies of eye color genetics in *Drosophila* by [39] to studies by Francis Crick et al. [40] that first implicated the genetic code occurred in triplets, as well as later studies that revealed unusual 4-base codons [41] and numerous other findings including those relating to the gram-negative envelope barrier function of *yfgL* [42–45].

"*Suppressor analysis*," the process of isolating, identifying suppressor mutations and their phenotypic [46–49], is also encompassed by several other related terminologies: "*Epistasis*" is the condition where the phenotype derived from a primary gene is modified by at least one secondary gene and in the process the phenotype is altered or suppressed. "*Pseudo-reversion*" refers to the fact that a particular phenotype is eliminated not by a simple back mutation, but by a secondary suppressor mutation. "*Tolerance acquisition*" may refer to primary mutations or secondary suppressor mutations. "*Compensatory mutation*" and "*rescue mutation*" also generally refer to secondary suppressor mutations. "*Chemical conditionality*" [42] is a subset of suppressor analysis studies where the primary mutation makes an organism susceptible to a particular chemical, and thereby suitable for selection of secondary suppressor mutations that counteract the sensitivity.

Suppressor mutations can be further classified as either "*interaction-*" or "*bypass-*" *suppressor mutations*. Interaction-suppressor mutations are gain-of-function mutations in proteins or their reaction products that physically interact with the mutant version of the primary protein or its reaction products (for example, the gene product of a temperature-sensitive allele where the primary mutation prevents the protein from interacting with its partner protein). A second class of suppressor mutations comprise bypass suppressor mutations. These suppressor mutations bypass the defects caused by the primary mutation by providing an alternative protein or pathway function, or eliminating such a protein or function, that thereby removes the stress caused by the primary mutation.

Primary *msbB* mutants in *Salmonella* have one or more defects in outer membrane barrier function that induce sensitivity to bile as well as a range of other chemical and environmental conditions [30]. This results in a wide range of bypass suppressor mutations that can be obtained. Selection of *msbB* suppressors in *Salmonella* has already identified several non-*yfgL* suppressors, including *somA* [30], *Suwwan* [31], *pmrA^C* [32], and *zwf* [33], three out of four of which (other than *pmrA^C*), are similar to *yfgL*, in that they are also deletion mutations that result in a gain in a gain-of-function (*see* Table 1). The chemical sensitivities induced by *msbB* mutation and the range of suppressor phenotypes are only known to occur in *Salmonella* and not in *E. coli* [30] and thus distinguish our studies from those on *E. coli*. Our understanding of differences in the outer membrane barrier function of *E. coli* and *Salmonella* will be advanced by these studies.

Other outer-membrane stress responses have been studied in *E. coli* [50–52] and suppressors have also been isolated, including sigma^E, a transcription factor [53] that leads to alterations in peptidoglycan [54–57]. Outer-membrane lipoproteins in *E. coli* are also required for the enzymes that synthesize peptidoglycan, which suggests that cell wall biogenesis requires components in both the inner and outer cell membranes [58, 59]. *sipB* is an outer-membrane permeability suppressor in both *E. coli* and *Salmonella* that have an F-plasmid [60] and might also potentially suppress the chemical conditionality of *msbB* lipidA mutants.

Below, we describe the methods we used for isolation and analysis of suppressor mutations in *msbB Salmonella*. While next-generation DNA sequencing offers an important alternative approach to elucidating suppressor mutations, the methods we provide have the benefits of (1) being applicable to high-throughput discovery of suppressor phenotypes, (2) specifically linking phenotype to genotype, and are especially useful for organisms for which there is no reference genome, (3) being applicable to the construction of strains suitable for use in humans, which have recombination and assembly requirements that go beyond DNA sequencing [15, 29], and (4) encompassing methods essential to understanding of microbial genetics and evolution, that are appropriate for learning and/or research settings.

2 Materials

2.1 Bacterial Strains, Plasmids, Phage, and Transposons

1. Bacterial strains: wild type *Salmonella* ATCC 14028, the attenuated strain VNP20009 (ATCC (202165; aka 41.2.9 or YS1646; [29]) and the unsuppressed *msbB Salmonella* strain YS8211 (*see* **Note 1**); ATCC 202026; [15] (American Type Culture Collection, Manassas, VA). *Salmonella* JR501 [61] TT58 (*ilv*-595::Tn*10*) and TT289 (*purE*::Tn*10*) are available from the *Salmonella* genetic stock center (Calgary, Canada; strain 1593) (*see* **Note 2**). *Escherichia coli* TOP10 is available from Invitrogen/Life Technologies (Grand Island, NY). All strains are stored frozen at −80 °C in 15 % glycerol.

2. Plasmids: pUC18 (Fisher Scientific, Waltham, MA) and pNK2883 ([62]; Nancy Kleckner, Harvard University, Cambridge, MA).

3. Tn*5* transpososome: EZ-Tn5 <Kan> (Epicenter, Madison, WI).

4. The phage: P22 (= mutant HT105/1*int201*; *Salmonella* Genetic Stock Center, Calgary, Canada).

2.2 Bacterial Media and Phage Diluent

1. Bacterial media: LB [63] which contains 1 % tryptone, 0.5 % yeast extract, and 1 % $NaCl_2$; or LB plates containing agar, LB-0 (LB no salt [29]), which contains of 1 % tryptone, 0.5 % yeast extract; or LB-0 plates containing agar, LB-0-EGTA [29] which consists of LB-0 with ethylene glycol-bis(β-aminoethyl ether)-N,N,N',N'-tetraacetic acid (EGTA, free acid) added as a sterile supplement to 3 mM from a 300 mM stock adjusted to pH 8.0 and autoclaved; or LB-0-EGTA plates containing agar, MSB (LB-0 with 2 mM $MgSO_4$ and 2 mM $CaCl_2$; [29]) adjusted to pH 7 using 1 N NaOH; or MSB plates containing agar, and MacConkey agar base (Difco) with added galactose (0.2 %). M9 minimal medium [64], used for auxotroph identification media pools, contains 0.5 % L-amino acids or 1 % D-L-amino acids, 0.5 % uracil or guanine, 0.5 % thymidine or adenosine. For Pool 7 (see below) solubility is achieved in 0.2 N sodium hydroxide (to dissolve tyrosine); all others in

hydrochloric acid up to 0.2 N made from stocks that are auto-claved for 10 min, cooled, and contain a few drops of added chloroform. To generate each petri plate pool (R. G. Lloyd, personal communication) as described below, add three drops to each petri plate, and add ~30 ml of M9 agar medium (held at 45 °C after autoclaving) to the same plate, mix, and let solidify. The pools consist of (1) arginine, histidine, methio-nine, proline (pH 5); (2) alanine, cysteine, glutamine, glycine (pH 3.5); (3) asparagine, isoleucine, lysine, uracil (pH 5.5); (4) adenosine, leucine, thymine, threonine (pH 5.5); (5) gua-nine, phenylalanine, tryptophan, tyrosine (pH 0.5); (6) ade-nosine, asparagine, glycine, histidine, tryptophan (pH 4.8); (7) alanine, lysine, proline, thymine, tyrosine (pH 10.5); (8) argi-nine, cysteine, phenylalanine, threonine, uracil (pH 1.2); and (9) glutamine, guanine, isoleucine(valine), leucine, methio-nine (pH 2). Plates used for most bacterial procedures contain 1.5 % agar, while 2.0 % is used for replica plating.

2. Antibiotics. Use as indicated: 50 μg/ml ampicillin (Amp_{50}), 20 μg/ml tetracycline (tet_{20}), and 20 μg/ml kanamycin (kan_{20}).

3. Gene induction agent: Isopropyl β-D-1-thiogalactopyranoside (IPTG) is used at 1 mM.

4. Phage diluent consists of 10 mM $MgSO_4$, 10 mM Tris pH 7.0.

2.3 Cancer Cells and Murine Tumor Models

1. Cancer cells: B16F10 and Cloudman S91M3 mouse mela-noma cells from the ATCC (Manassas, VA) were cultured in Corning plastic tissue culture flasks in Dulbecco's Modified Eagle Medium (DMEM) supplemented with heat-inactivated fetal bovine serum (10 % vol/vol; Gibco/Life Technologies, Grand Island, NY).

2. Mice: C57BL/6 and DBA/2J mice are available from Jackson Laboratories (Bar Harbor, ME); C57B6 mice are compatible hosts for B16F10 melanoma cells and DBA/2J mice are com-patible hosts for Cloudman S91M3 melanoma cells.

2.4 DNA Manipulations

1. PCR: BioMix Red (Bioline, Taunton, MA).

2. Agarose gels: DNA is separated using 0.9 % agarose in tris-acetate–ethylenediaminetetraacetic acid (EDTA) (TAE) buffer consisting of 40 mM Tris, 20 mM acetic acid, and 1 mM EDTA with 1:10,000 of a 1 % solution of ethidium bromide added for visualization under ultraviolet light.

3. Buffers: Tris-EDTA (TE) buffer consists of 10 mM Tris adjusted to pH 8.0 with HCl and 1 mM EDTA. Sodium-saline-citrate (SSC) buffer is made from a 10× stock of SSC consisting of 1.5 M sodium chloride 150 mM tri-sodium citrate with the pH adjusted to 7.0 using HCl.

4. Isolation of genomic DNA: From a modified procedure [65]: the cell-suspension buffer contains 10 mM Tris–HCl (pH 8.0) with 2.5 mg/ml lysozyme, 1 mM NaEDTA, and 0.035 M sucrose. Lysis solution contains 100 mM Tris (pH 8.0), 0.3 M NaCl, 20 mM EDTA, 2 % SDS (w/v); add 2 % β-mercaptoethanol (BME) and 100 μg/ml proteinase K, and 0.5 volumes of 5 M sodium perchlorate just prior to use in order to avoid precipitates. 10 % SDS (sodium dodecyl sulfate) 20 mg/ml proteinase K, phenol–chloroform–isoamyl alcohol solution (25:24:1), 70 and 100 % isopropanol, 70 and 100 % ethanol, 3 M sodium acetate pH 5.2, and glycogen are also used where indicated.

5. Restriction enzymes: New England Biolabs (Beverly, MA).

6. DNA isolation from gels: Gene Clean II (MP Biochemicals, Santa Ana, CA).

7. Identification of transposon insertions sites: GenomeWalker purchased from Clonetech (Mountain View, CA).

8. Cloning PCR products: TA cloning kit (Invitrogen/Life Technologies, Grand Island, NY).

2.5 Other Equipment   Scienceware® replica plater for nutrient plates (Sigma-Aldrich Z363391, St. Louis, MO) and velveteen squares (Sigma-Aldrich Z363405) may be used for "double velvet" and "triple velvet" replica plating [47, 66]; our labs use velvet fabric from a fabric supply store sterilized by autoclaving.

3 Methods

3.1 Isolation and Initial Characterization of Spontaneous msbB Suppressor Mutants

1. Streak *msbB Salmonella* strain YS8211 from a frozen stock (in 15 % glycerol) on an MSB [29] agar plate and incubate overnight at 37 °C to obtain isolated colonies (*see* **Note 1**). Inoculate individual colonies in separate tubes of MSB broth and incubate until they reach an OD_{600} of 0.100. Hold cultures on ice until all cultures reached the desired OD (*see* **Note 3**).

2. Prepare serial dilutions from 10^{-1} to 10^{-7} in MSB broth and hold them on ice (*see* **Note 4**). Plate 10^{-3} final dilutions onto LB-0-EGTA and galactose MacConkey agar plates, 10^{-4} final dilution onto LB agar, 10^{-7} final dilutions on MSB agar plates and incubate overnight at 37 °C to determine the frequency of LB, EGTA, or MacConkey-resistant cells in the population.

3. Select a random subset of different-sized colonies arising on LB, EGTA, or MacConkey media on MSB agar plates, restreak to the same media and incubate overnight at 37 °C.

4. Patch ten colonies of each onto an MSB agar master plate and incubate overnight at 37 °C for use in replica plating. This tests

for the genetic stability of the suppressor mutation (*see* **Note 5**).

5. Replica-plate patches of cells from an MSB agar master plate onto a new MSB agar plate, creating a "first velvet" master plate [47], and then replica-plate the "first velvet" master plate (without incubation) onto MSB agar (creating a "second velvet" master plate), as well as EGTA, and MacConkey plates. Then, replica-plate the unincubated "second velvet" MSB master plate onto LB media, and incubate all plates overnight at 37 °C to determine the frequency of LB-, EGTA-, or MacConkey-resistant colonies from the isolated clones in order to determine their genetic stability (*see* **Note 6**).

6. Interpret the individual clones as follows: if all ten patched colonies have the same suppressor phenotype then the genetic mutation can be assumed to be stable; if only a portion retain the suppressor phenotype, the clones should be considered to be unstable. Tabulate the relative growth of each of the potential clones on the different media using a –, +, ++, or +++ notation (*see* **Note 7**).

3.2 Genetic Identification of Spontaneous Mutations by Transposon Linkage and Further Characterization

3.2.1 Preparation of Electrocompetent Salmonella (See **Note 8**)

1. Inoculate a 2 ml culture of MSB media from a single colony on a fresh overnight MSB plate of a *Salmonella* strain and incubate at 37 °C with shaking at 200 rpm overnight.

2. The following morning add 1 ml of culture to ~100 ml of pre-warmed MSB media at 37 °C and incubate with shaking at 200 rpm until the culture density reaches OD_{600} 0.6; usually 2–3 h (*see* **Note 9**).

3. Place the culture on ice to rapidly cool for 15 min, and then transfer 40 ml to prechilled 50 ml Falcon blue-top #2089 centrifuge tubes.

4. Using a prechilled rotor, pellet the bacteria at $8000 \times g$ for 10 min at 4 °C.

5. Pour off the supernatant into a bio-hazard container for disposal.

6. Resuspend the pellet in 4 ml sterile 1 % glycerol in ultra-pure water (*see* **Note 10**) pre-chilled to 4 °C using a pre-chilled serological pipette.

7. Transfer 0.5 ml of the culture (up to 16 tubes for 16 independent transformations) to pre-chilled 1.5 ml micro-fuge tubes (Eppendorf).

8. Using a pre-chilled micro-fuge placed in a refrigerator or cold-room, pellet the bacteria at $8000 \times g$ for 1 min at 4 °C.

9. Aspirate off the supernatant into a bio-hazard container for disposal.

10. Add 1.0 ml of sterile 1 % glycerol in ultra-pure water pre-chilled to 4 °C.

11. Using a pre-chilled P1000 micro-pipette tip and a P1000 micropipettor, resuspend the pellet by pipetting up and down until you have generated a homogeneous suspension.

12. Centrifuge as described in **step 8** and discard the supernatant as in **step 9**.

13. Repeat **steps 10–12** two additional times.

14. Add 1.0 ml of sterile 10 % glycerol in ultra-pure water pre-chilled to 4 °C.

15. Using a pre-chilled P1000 micro-pipette tip and a P1000 micropipettor, resuspend the pellet by pipetting up and down until a homogeneous suspension is generated.

16. Repeat **steps 10** and **11** one additional time.

17. Resuspend the bacterial pellet in 40 μl 10 % sterile glycerol in ultrapure water.

18. Freeze at −80 °C.

3.2.2 Determination of Electrocompetent Salmonella Transformation Efficiency

1. Thaw the electrocompetent *Salmonella* on ice.

2. Prepare a transformation standard using DNA of a known concentration purchased from a vendor (e.g., pUC18, Fisher Scientific S66765), and adjust the concentration to 1.0 ng/μl.

3. Prechill a sterile 1.0 mm electroporation cuvette (Bio-Rad) on ice.

4. Pipette 1 μl of the 1 ng/μl plasmid into the electro-competent cells using a sterile prechilled extra-long gel loading type tip.

5. Set the micro-pipettor to 41 μl and gently pipette the entire volume up and down in order to mix.

6. Pipette the cell mixture into the electroporation cuvette (*see* **Note 11**).

7. Set the electroporator to 1.7 kV, 200 Ω and 25 μFD (*see* **Note 8**).

8. Pulse the cuvette and note the time constant (*see* **Note 12**).

9. Remove the cuvette from the electroporator chamber and immediately add 960 μl warm (~30 °C) MSB medium.

10. Using a P1000 transfer as much of the material as possible to a 15 ml polypropylene tube, and remove the remaining material with a gel-loader tip to the same tube.

11. Allow the bacteria to recover for 1 h at 37 °C with shaking.

12. Perform ten-fold serial dilutions to 10^{-3} into 1 % glycerol (*see* **Note 13**) and plate 100 μl to individual petri plates containing the appropriate antibiotic maker (e.g., 50 μg/ml ampicillin) for pUC18.

13. Incubate the plates at 37 °C in ambient air overnight.

14. Count the colonies of plates where there are between 30 and 300 colony forming units (CFU).

15. Based on the number of colonies, the dilution factor, amount of cells plated (0.1 ml) and the total volume (1.0 ml), extrapolate the number of antibiotic-resistant bacteria per nanogram and multiply by 1000 to determine the number of transformants per microgram. Transformation efficiencies should be greater than 5×10^7 (preferably greater than 1×10^8); if this level is not achieved then re-perform the competent cell procedure (Subheadings 3.2.1 and 3.2.2).

3.2.3 Generation of a Tn10 Transposon Library

1. Electroporate pNK2883 (amp^R but tet_{20}^S) into wild-type ATCC 14028 *Salmonella* and plate on LB-amp$_{50}$ to generate 14028 pNK2883 (*see* **Note 14**).

2. Grow a shaking culture of 14028 pNK2883 at 37 °C to an OD_{600} of 0.400 in LB-Amp$_{50}$ broth and then split the cultures into two, adding 1 mM IPTG to one culture to induce transposition of Tn10 into the chromosome. After adding the IPTG (and not adding it to the control), incubate the cultures for 2 h on a shaker at 37 °C and place the cultures on ice.

3. Create a dilution series (in ice-cold LB-amp$_{50}$ broth) to determine the CFU/ml of tetracycline-resistant colonies in each culture by plating the dilutions onto LB-tet$_{20}$ agar and incubating overnight at 37 °C in order to confirm that the transposition is IPTG-dependent and determine the number of CFU/ml; retain the serial dilutions on ice overnight.

4. After demonstrating that transposition was IPTG-dependent and calculating the CFU/ml of the tetracycline-resistant colonies in the culture, plate enough colonies to screen at least five times the number of genes present in the organism (*see* **Note 15**).

3.2.4 Genetic Identification of Spontaneous Mutations by Transposon Linkage and Further Characterization; Analysis of Transposon Library by Identification of Different Auxotrophs

1. Confirm that the library generated at least 0.5 % auxotrophy in various biosynthetic pathways by double-velvet replica plating a portion of the library (at least 1000 colonies) onto M9 minimal medium [64] and LB agar [63] (*see* **Note 16**).

2. Patch any colonies growing on LB (no antibiotic) agar but not M9 agar onto an LB agar plate to create a master plate containing a positive control prototrophic strain (ATCC 14028 wild type) and a negative control auxotroph (e.g., TT58 (*ilv*-595::Tn10) or TT289 (*purE*::Tn10)). Generate a double-velvet replica-plate series that includes LB agar, M9 minimal agar, and M9 minimal agar with combinations of the following amino acids in the pool table below:

Table 2
Amino acid and nucleotide pools for determining auxotrophy

	Pool 1	Pool 2	Pool 3	Pool 4	Pool 5
Pool 6	Histidine	Glycine (or serine)	Asparagine	Adenosine	Tryptophan (or aromatic if only grows on pool 5, but not pool 6)
Pool 7	Proline	Alanine	Lysine	Thymine	Tyrosine
Pool 8	Arginine (or pyrimidine if only grows on pool 8, but not 1)	Cysteine	Uracil	Threonine	Phenylalanine
Pool 9	Methioinine	Glutamine	Isoleucine/valine	Leucine	Guanine

3. Use the following table (Table 2) to determine which type of auxotroph was obtained where the type of auxotroph listed in the box indicates that the organism grew on the pools listed in the corresponding row and column.

   If at least 0.5 % auxotrophs, representing mutants in various pathways, are obtained, then proceed to the next step: pooling of the Tn*10* library. If the library does not produce minimum 0.5 % auxotrophy, repeat the transposon mutagenesis.

4. Pool the Tn*10* library by adding MSB broth to the surface of the plates and aseptically suspend colonies from the agar surface in the broth using a sterilized glass spreader and/or inoculating loop.

5. Once colonies from all the plates have been suspended, transfer the LB broth culture to a sterile flask; this is the *transposon library*.

6. Mix well and create several frozen-stock aliquots in LB broth with a final concentration of 15 % glycerol (*see* **Note 17**).

3.2.5 Titering P22 Phage, Preparing P22 Phage Stocks and Phage Lysates from Donor Strains

1. P22 phage is usually supplied at 10^{10}–10^{11} PFU/ml; this procedure both determines the actual number of phage and expands the amount of the phage.

2. Dilute phage (~10^{-6} to 10^{-7}) into 10 mM MgSO$_4$ 10 mM Tris pH 7.0.

3. Add an aliquot (e.g., 0.1 ml) to ~0.1 ml P22-sensitive cells such as ATCC 14028 from a log phase culture (*see* **Note 18**).

4. Add soft agar overlay of ~3 ml, 0.5 % agar in LB.

5. Mix and pour onto a LB plate (pre-warmed to 37 °C) and incubate at 37 °C overnight.

6. Count the plates with between 30 and 300 plaque-forming units (PFU)/plate and extrapolate the total number of plaques obtained based on the number of plaques per plate, the dilution factor for that plate and the volume of phage plated, which represents the *phage titer*.

7. To generate the new phage stock, dilute an overnight culture of a P22-sensitive strain 1:5 into fresh LB, add P22 phage $\sim 5 \times 10^6$/ml.

8. Grow at 37 °C, 5–18 h.

9. Add a few drops chloroform to eliminate bacteria, vortex 10 s every 3 min for a total of 12 min and let stand for ~10 min.

10. Centrifuge for ~$8000 \times g$ 10 min.

11. Carefully remove the supernatant, avoiding the bottom of the tube (supernatant = new P22 stock).

12. Check to ensure there are no surviving bacteria by spotting a drop of the new P22 stock onto LB media and incubating overnight.

13. If bacteria are found, repeat the chloroform treatment and spot check if any bacteria grow until none are detected.

14. The *new phage stock* can then be titered as described above.

15. A *phage lysate* that will contain transducing phages with the desired selectable genetic markers is prepared using a donor strain or mixed-donor strains (as described below) that contain the genetic marker(s), by repeating **steps 7–13** above.

*3.2.6 Creation of Phage-P22-Transducing Tn10 Library (See **Note 19**)*

Dilute the mixed bacterial Tn*10* library in fresh LB broth to an OD_{600} of 0.100 and grow to an OD_{600} of 0.400.

1. Add 5.0×10^6 PFU of phage P22 and incubate for 5–18 h on a test-tube rotator at 37 °C and then add 40 μl chloroform per 1 ml (*see* **Note 20**).

2. Vortex for 10 s every 3 min, for a total of 12 min.

3. Pellet the cell debris at maximum speed in a clinical centrifuge.

4. Carefully transfer the supernatant (*phage lysate*) to another tube without pipetting any of the cell debris at the bottom of the tube; this is the phage-*P22-transducing* Tn*10 library lysate*.

3.2.7 Genetic Mapping of Spontaneous Suppressor Mutations by Linkage of Transposons to a Suppressor Mutation

1. Inoculate a single colony of the suppressor strain in MSB broth and incubate on a rotating platform at 150 RPM until an OD_{600} of 0.400 is reached (*see* **Note 21**).

2. Begin phage transduction by adding an aliquot of the P22 transducing-phage lysate with a multiplicity of infection (MOI) of ~1 (PFU/ml) to 20 (CFU/ml) ratio and allow to stand for 10 min at room temp. Some selections such as Kan^R require

~2 h non-selection at 37 °C prior to selection conditions in order to express the antibiotic resistance.

3. Aliquot dilutions onto LB-0-tet$_{20}$-agar plates (*see* **Note 22**) and add 3 ml of 0.5 % soft agar overlay, mixing well by gently moving the plate back and forth. Incubate the soft-agar plates for 1–2 days at 37 °C (*see* **Note 23**).

4. Patch colonies (including positive and negative controls) onto LB-0-tet$_{20}$ agar and incubate these master plates overnight at 37 °C.

5. Double velvet-replica-plate (as described above in Subheading 3.3.1) onto LB-0, EGTA, and galactose MacConkey media and then triple velvet-replica-plate onto LB agar to assess the presence of the unsuppressed *msbB* phenotype (i.e., sensitivity to EGTA, MacConkey, or LB agar) is restored in any patches.

6. Restreak any patches that have an unsuppressed *msbB* phenotype to isolate pure colonies.

7. Make a new master plate as described in Subheading 3.3.3 on LB no-salt agar and replica plate to confirm that the Tn*10* is linked to the wild-type version of the suppressor gene.

3.2.8 Creation of Strains with Tn10 Linked to Wild Type and Mutant Alleles of the Suppressor Gene

1. Inoculate single colonies of each strain with a Tn*10* linked to a suppressor gene in MSB broth and grow overnight at 37 °C.

2. Generate a phage lysate as described above in Subheading 3.2.5.

3. Perform transduction as described in Subheading 3.2.7.

4. Patch 20–100 transductants derived from each strain (the higher the number, the more accurate the frequency) onto LB-0 agar, incubate overnight, and double-velvet replicate plate onto media related to the suppressor phenotype, such as EGTA or galactose-MacConkey agar.

5. Record the co-transduction frequency data (the frequency of transductants losing the suppressor phenotype) to determine the approximate distance between the Tn*10* and the suppressor mutation.

6. Estimate how close the Tn*10* is to the suppressor mutation using the formula: co-transduction frequency = (1 − (distance between two markers in Kb)/(length of transducing particle genome) (*see* **Notes 24** and **25**).

3.2.9 Cloning msbB Suppressor Mutations

1. In order to isolate genomic DNA using a strain that has a Tn*10* linked to a suppressor mutation, pellet a 25 ml overnight culture and discard the supernatant.

2. Resuspend the cell pellet in 3.75 ml of cell suspension buffer containing 2.5 mg/ml of lysozyme and incubate at room temperature for 15 min.

3. Add 5.5 ml of warm (~30 °C) lysis solution.

4. Add an equal volume of phenol–chloroform–isoamyl alcohol, mix for 5–10 min, centrifuge for 10 min at $8000 \times g$. Transfer the aqueous phase to a new tube. Repeat this step until there is no white protein interface left.

5. Add an equal volume of chloroform–isoamyl alcohol and extract two to three times until no white protein interface is observed. Transfer the aqueous phase to a new tube.

6. Precipitate the DNA by adding 1/10 volume of 3 M sodium acetate and mixing well by inverting the tube, add two volumes of 100 % ethanol and mix gently.

7. Spool DNA with a glass rod by swirling and turning the rod until the two phases are mixed.

8. Gently squeeze out the excess EtOH on a beaker wall and rinse twice by immersing in 70 % ethanol for 5 min.

9. Air-dry for 30 min and resuspend DNA in 2.5 ml TE buffer.

10. Quantitate the DNA concentration using a spectrophotometer.

11. Perform a *Sau*3AI partial digestion of genomic DNA by adding 75 µl of genomic DNA (approx. 2 µg), 15 µl of 10× digestion buffer, and 60 µl of de-ionized water to an Eppendorf tube (with 150 µl total volume).

12. Aliquot this solution into 1 tube of 30 µl, 3 tubes of 20 µl, and 1 tube of 10 µl. Label the tubes 1, 2, 3, 4, and 5. Put the tubes on ice.

13. To test tube #1, add 5 units of *Sau*3AI per 1 µg of DNA. Mix well by pipetting up and down, but do not vortex.

14. Perform serial dilutions by pipetting 10 µl from tube 1, to tube 2, mixing well, and then transferring 10 µl to tube 3, mixing well, and transferring 10 µl to tube 4, mixing well, and then transferring 10 µl to tube 5.

15. Incubate for 15 min at 37 °C and immediately place the reactions on ice after incubation. Then quickly add 0.5 µl of 0.5 M EDTA to kill the reaction.

16. Run a gel with loading all of the samples into the wells. Look for which concentration best produces a bright smear near the size of the fragments that you would like to clone into the plasmid. We recommend 5–10 Kb fragments, which can be easily sequenced (*see* **Note 26**).

17. Scale up the reaction to digest 5 µg of genomic DNA, using the same optimum stoichiometry and enzyme concentration as described above.

18. Run a gel of the optimized *Sau*3AI-digested genomic DNA and cut the bands of the desired size out of the gel using a clean razor blade or scalpel. Do this quickly to minimize mutation by the UV light (*see* **Note 27**). Use the Gene Clean II Kit (MP Biomedicals) following manufacturer's protocol for purification of the agarose-separated *Sau*3AI partial digest.

19. Ligate the genomic DNA library into the pre-digested and dephosphorylated (to prevent re-ligation of empty vector) cloning vector (encoding an antibiotic resistance other than tetracycline) with *Bgl*II, *Bam*HI, or another enzyme reacting with sticky ends compatible with *Sau*3AI and perform a ligation, using the optimum ratio of three molecules of digested insert for every one molecule of digested vector (*see* **Note 28**).

20. Transform the library into chemically-competent TOP10 *E. coli* using heat shock and plate the cells onto LB with selection of Tet^R and another antibiotic-resistance marker found on the vector (e.g., ampicillin) in order to simultaneously select for both the Tn*10* and the antibiotic resistance gene on the vector.

21. Sequence the DNA inserts in positive clones using universal primers for vector and transposon.

22. Compare the DNA sequences from the wild-type and mutant libraries in order to reveal the suppressor mutation.

23. Determine if the suppressor mutation is dominant or recessive by complementing the mutant using the same region of DNA cloned from the wild type, by PCR, and observe phenotypes related to suppression. If the un-suppressed phenotype is restored (i.e., EGTA^S), then the wild type allele is dominant. If the strain is still suppressed with both wild type and mutant alleles, then the mutant is dominant, which can be further confirmed by electroporating the mutant version of the gene into the unsuppressed *msbB* mutant and evaluating the suppressor phenotype (i.e., EGTA^R) as described above.

3.3 Isolation of Transposon-Induced Suppressor Mutations Resulting in Resistance to CO_2

When VNP20009 is plated in standard media such as LB and incubated under 5 % atmospheric CO_2, the plating efficiency is dramatically reduced compared to non-CO_2 conditions (*see* **Note 29**). Karsten et al. [33] have shown that deletion of the *zwf* gene suppresses sensitivity to CO_2.

3.3.1 Transformation of Electrocompetent Salmonella to Generate a Tn5 Library

1. Thaw the electro-competent *Salmonella* on ice.

2. Thaw the Tn*5* transpososome on ice.

3. Prechill a 1.0 mm electroporation cuvette on ice.

4. Pipette 1 μl of the transpososome into the electro-competent cells using a pre-chilled extra-long gel loading type tip.

5. Set the micro-pipettor to 41 μl and gently pipette the entire volume up and down in order to mix.

6. Pipette the cell–transpososome mixture into a 1 mm electroporation cuvette (*see* **Note 11**).

7. Set the electroporator to 1.7 kV, 200 Ω and 25 μF if using VNP20009 (*see* **Note 8**). Pulse the cuvette and note the time constant (*see* **Note 12**).

8. Remove the cuvette from the electroporator chamber and immediately add 1 ml warm (~30 °C) MSB media.

9. Using a P1000, transfer as much of the material as possible to a 15 ml polypropylene tube, and remove the remaining material with a gel-loader tip to the same tube.

10. Allow the bacteria to recover for 1 h at 37 °C with shaking.

3.3.2 Plating and Expansion of the Salmonella Tn5 Library

1. Based on a typical transformation rate of 1×10^8 transformants/μg of supercoiled pUC18 as described above, place the entire library in equal amounts on three, 150 mm petri plates with LB-0 agar medium and antibiotic (e.g., 20 μg/ml kanamycin for Tn5), by placing ~333 μl on of the plates and spreading with a sterilized glass spreader (*see* **Note 30**).

2. Incubate overnight at 37 °C.

3. Measure a 2×2 cm subsection of the plate using a ruler and count the number of colonies within it (*see* **Note 31**).

4. Flood each of the plates with 5 ml of liquid LB-0 kan_{20}.

5. Using a sterile glass spreader, dislodge all of the colonies on each of the plates.

6. Using a 5 ml serological pipette, remove the liquid from each of the pates and combine into one 50 ml sterile tube.

7. Estimate the amount of total liquid and add sufficient sterile 80 % glycerol/water to bring the concentration of glycerol to 15 %.

8. Freeze the library in 1 ml aliquots at −80 °C.

3.3.3 Plating the Salmonella Tn5 Library for Suppressor Mutants and Determination of the Plating Efficiency

1. A ~10 μl sub-sample of a frozen vial may be obtained without thawing the vial by scraping the top of the vial with a sterile weighing spatula or sterile wooden applicator and quickly transferring it to a sterile micro-fuge tube for it to thaw (*see* **Note 32**).

2. Perform ten-fold serial dilutions down to 10^{-8} and place 100 μl per plate to determine the CFU concentration.

3. Perform a CO_2-selection experiment by culturing a tenfold dilution series that will yield between 30 and 300 colony forming units (CFU)/plate in duplicate.

4. Place one set of plates at 37 °C in ambient air and incubate overnight.

5. Place the other set of plates at 37 °C in 5 % CO_2 and incubate overnight.

6. Count the colonies on plates with between 30 and 300 colony forming units (CFU)/plate and extrapolate the total number of colonies obtained under each of the two conditions based on the number of colonies per plate, the dilution factor for that plate and the amount of cells plated.

7. Divide the number of total colonies obtained under CO_2 conditions by the total number of colonies obtained under ambient air conditions in order to determine the plating efficiency or percent survival under CO_2 conditions (*see* **Note 33**).

8. The Tn5 library cells grown under CO_2 conditions represent the first round of selection and may contain both spontaneous and Tn5-induced mutations (*see* **Note 34**). These bacteria are used for subsequent rounds of purification and as donors cells for phage transduction described below.

3.3.4 Enriching Tn5-Based msbB Suppressor Mutations Over Spontaneous Mutations by Phage Transduction

1. Inoculate the CO_2-selected Tn5 library (as described in Sub-headings 3.3.2 and 3.3.3) in MSB broth and grow overnight in a shaking incubator at 37 °C.

2. Generate a phage lysate as described above in Sub-heading 3.2.5.

3. Perform a transduction to move the Tn5 library into a CO_2-sensitive strain as described in Sub-heading 3.2.7 with the following modifications (**steps 4–12** below).

4. Pre-absorb the phage by incubating them for 15 min at 37 °C.

5. Begin washing the bacteria to remove un-adsorbed phage by pelleting them in a micro-fuge for 1 min at full speed (e.g., $17,000 \times g$).

6. Resuspend the bacteria in 1 mL LB-0 broth + 3 mM EGTA (*see* **Note 35**).

7. Incubate at room temperature for 5 min.

8. Pellet the bacteria in a micro-fuge 1 min at full speed (e.g., $15,000 \times g$).

9. Repeat wash (**steps 6–9**) two additional times to remove un-adsorbed phage (*see* **Note 36**).

10. After the final wash resuspend bacteria in 1 mL LB-0 + 3 mM EGTA. Some selections including Kan^R require ~2 h non-selection at 37 °C conditions prior to selection conditions in order to express the antibiotic resistance. Plate 50 μL, 200 μL and the ~750 μl remainder to LB-0 with 20 μg/mL kanamycin

(or other appropriate antibiotic depending upon the genetic marker used).

11. Incubate the plates at 37 °C.

12. Bacterial colonies should be visible the next day but may take longer for some strains.

3.3.5 Analysis of Transposon Linkage to CO$_2$ Resistance

1. Determine three individual colony linkages to CO$_2$ resistance by transducing from three individual donor colonies from Sub-heading 3.3.4 as described in Sub-heading 3.2.7 to generate multiple-phage transduction-derived antibiotic resistant colonies from each of the three original colonies. *See* Sub-heading 3.2.8 above on linkage distances; as these are insertional mutations they should be 100 % linked.

2. Using a sterilized needle or sterile wooden toothpics, grid individual colonies as patches an on antibiotic plate and allow growth at 37 °C overnight in ambient air.

3. Perform the double-velvet replica technique to generate two identical plates (*see* Subheading 3.1 above).

4. Incubate one plate at 37 °C in air and the other in 37 °C under 5 % CO$_2$ overnight.

5. Score the plates for the number of patches with uninhibited growth under CO$_2$ as being CO$_2$ resistant.

6. Linkage is confirmed by the complete correlation of the presence of the Tn5 insertions with CO$_2$ resistance (resistant colonies/total colonies = 100 %).

3.3.6 Determine Plating Efficiency of CO$_2$-Resistant Clones

1. Pick an individual CO$_2$-resistant colony from a replica plate experiment and inoculate LB-0 medium and grow over-night at 37 °C with shaking in ambient air.

2. Plate serial dilutions of the bacteria onto LB-0 agar down to 10^{-6} using 100 µl of the serially-diluted material and incubate one plate at 37 °C in air and the other in 37 °C under 5 % CO$_2$ overnight.

3. Score the plates for the number of colonies following CO$_2$ incubation where the colonies have the same approximate size (i.e., not significantly smaller) as those grown under incubation in air as being resistant to CO$_2$.

4. Divide the number of CO$_2$-resistant colonies by the total number of colonies grown on air to obtain the percentage of CO$_2$-resistant colonies, also referred to as the plating efficiency.

3.3.7 Determination of the Chromosomal Insertion Site of the Tn5 Transposon

1. An alternative to constructing a plasmid-based DNA library containing the Tn-insertion (e.g., Tn5 or Tn10) and it's selectable marker, which is thereby used to identify the presence of the Tn (*see* Sub-heading 3.2.9) is to use the known sequence

of the Tn insertion itself as an anchor site for PCR of the unknown, adjacent upstream and downstream flanking sites in which the Tn is generating an insertion [67].

3.3.8   Purification of Genomic DNA from CO_2-Resistant Clones with Tn5 Insertions Linked to Resistance

3.3.9   Construction of Adaptor-Ligated Genomic DNA Fragments

1. A pool of adaptor-ligated genomic DNA fragments is constructed using a GenomeWalker Universal Kit (Clontech, Mountain View, CA). The kit comes with a complete set of instructions and a variety of controls from which our brief laboratory protocol is derived.

2. Digest 2.5 μg genomic DNA with *Eco*RV, and 2.5 μg genomic DNA with *Pvu*II, to completion (usually overnight) in a 100 μl reaction order to generate blunt ends.

3. Following digestion, begin purifying the DNA using an equal volume of phenol–chloroform–isoamyl alcohol by vortexing for 1 min.

4. Using a microfuge set to high speed (e.g., $17,000 \times g$), centrifuge the phenol-containing sample to separate the aqueous and organic phases.

5. Transfer the upper aqueous phase to a new centrifuge tube and add 100 μl of chloroform/isoamyl alcohol.

6. Vortex 1 min and then centrifuge for 1 min at high speed.

7. Transfer the upper aqueous phase to a new micro-fuge tube.

8. Add 0.1 volume of 3 M sodium acetate, 1 μl of 20 mg/ml glycogen and then precipitate the DNA by adding two volumes of 100 % ice-cold ethanol.

9. Vortex briefly and then centrifuge for 10 min at high speed.

10. Carefully aspirate off the supernatant leaving the small white DNA/glycogen pellet at the bottom.

11. Add 1.0 ml of 70 % ethanol and vortex briefly.

12. Centrifuge for 5 min at high speed.

13. Carefully aspirate off the supernatant, leaving the small white DNA/glycogen pellet at the bottom.

14. Allow the pellet to dry by leaving the cap off while the tube sits in a 37 °C heat block.

15. Dissolve the pellet in 20 μl sterile dH_2O.

16. For each of the blunt-end enzyme-digested DNA fragment pools, set up an adaptor ligation containing 4 μl of digested, purified DNA to a fresh 0.5-ml tube.

17. For each reaction add 1.9 μl GenomeWalker Adaptor (25 μM), 1.6 μl 10× ligation buffer and 0.5 μl T4 ligase (6 units/μl) and incubate at 16 °C overnight.

18. Stop the reactions at 70 °C for 5 min and then add 72 μl of TE (pH 7.5) and briefly vortex.

19. Based upon the sequence of the transposon used, design nested-insertion specific PCR primers with a G/C of 40–60 % and a length of at least 26 bp. Nested primers can be designed to amplify both flanking sequences. The Clontech GenomeWalker primers are also nested and have *Sal*I, *Mlu*I, *Srf*I, *Sma*I, and *Xma*I sites to facilitate cloning following PCR, or TA cloning (Invitrogen) may also be used.

20. Perform a hotstart PCR reaction using the outer adaptor primer and outer transposon primer for each of the 5′ and 3′ transposon ends and each of the fragment pools.

21. To eliminate spurious PCR products, use 1 μl of the first PCR reaction to perform a second PCR reaction with the inner set of nested primers for each of the 5′ and 3′ transposon ends and each of the fragment pools.

22. Run 5 μl of the PCR reaction in a 1 % agarose gel in TAE buffer in order to determine the presence of a PCR product from the second, inner-nested PCR.

23. Using standard cloning techniques, clone the positive PCR products and determine the DNA sequence in order to verify the presence of the transposon sequence and the site of its insertion.

3.4 In Vivo Analysis of Antitumor Efficacy

3.4.1 Cultivation and Implantation of Cancer Cells

1. Culture melanoma cells in Corning plastic tissue-culture flasks in DMEM nutrient medium supplemented with fetal bovine serum (10 % vol/vol) (Gibco/Life Technologies, Grand Island, NY).

2. Implant 5×10^5 B16F10 cells subcutaneously into the left shoulder region of C57B6 mice (Jackson Laboratories, Bar Harbor, Maine); C57B6 mice are compatible hosts for B16F10 melanoma cells.

3. Implant 5×10^5 Cloudman S91M3 cells subcutaneously into the left shoulder region of DBA/2J mice (Jackson Laboratories, Bar Harbor, Maine); DBA/2J mice are compatible hosts for Cloudman S91M3 melanoma cells.

3.4.2 Treatment of Tumor-Bearing Mice with Genetically-Engineered Salmonella

1. Obtain *Salmonella* from LB agar plates with a platinum bacterial loop.

2. Dilute bacteria to $OD_{600} = 0.05$ (~2×10^7 CFU/ml) in fresh Luria broth and grow overnight at 37 °C with gentle shaking.

3. The next day dilute again to $OD_{600} = 0.05$ into appropriate growth medium and grow at 37 °C to $OD_{600} = 0.8$ (~4×10^8 CFU).

4. Dilute bacteria into sterile H_2O or saline solution and, depending on the nature of the experiment, inject into mice intravenously (iv) via the tail vein or intraperitoneally (ip) at levels from 10^0 to 10^9 CFU/mouse; 2×10^6 CFU/mouse is a typical dose for VNP20009.

5. At designated times, sacrifice the animals, remove the tumors and livers, and weigh them.

6. Remove a central portion of the tumor and prepare it for microscopy.

7. Homogenize the remainder of the tumor in five volumes of LB broth per gram wet weight of tissue.

8. Quantitate the bacteria by serial dilution on LB agar plates, incubating for 1–3 days, 37 °C, and counting colonies.

*3.4.3 Evaluation of Antitumor Activity of Genetically-Engineered Salmonella (See **Note 37**)*

1. Begin measurements of tumor growth using calipers when tumors become palpable.

2. Follow tumor growth by periodic caliper measurements over the length of the experiment.

3. Euthanize the animals when the tumors reach a size predetermined by the institutional animal-welfare committee, e.g., 1000 mm^3, or should they became moribund.

4. Compute tumor volume by the formula: $L \times W \times H \times 0.5236 = mm^3$.

4   Notes

1. It is essential that when working with YS8211 or other unsuppressed *msbB Salmonella* strains, that MSB medium is used for propagation. Furthermore, several representative colonies from the original stock should be independently assessed for their phenotype as described by Murray et al. [30] which includes growth on MSB, sensitivity to salt, bile, EGTA and CO_2, using the replica-plating technique (e.g., [66]), as described in Sub-heading 3.1.

2. *Salmonella* are biosafety-level 2 (BSL-2) organisms. BSL-2 practices should be followed. Biosafety guidelines are available at the Centers for Disease Control website (http://www.cdc.gov/biosafety/publications/bmbl5/index.htm).

3. At an OD_{600} of 0.100, *Salmonella* has about ~5.0×10^7 CFU/ml.

4. Do not perform dilutions in PBS, as *msbB Salmonella* will not survive.

5. The master plate should include positive (wild-type and known suppressor strains) and negative controls (simple (unsuppressed) *msbB* mutant).

6. The double- and triple-velvet techniques are required to detect many growth defects that are not apparent using single-velvet replica plating. EGTA, MacConkey, and LB sensitivity are not observed using single-velvet replica plating and LB sensitivity is not observed using double-velvet replica plating. Agar plates for replica plating should be made with 2 % (not 1.5 %) agar. The plates should either be air- or incubator-dried until creases are visible on the surface of the agar. A completely smooth surface on an agar plate indicates that it is not ready for replica plating.

7. All of the *msbB* suppressors yield an intermediate phenotype—none restore the phenotype of wild type to *msbB Salmonella*. The various suppressor strains should be grouped based on similar phenotypes. Presumably similar phenotypes arise from mutation in the same, or convergent, pathways. Frozen stocks should be made, immediately after strain creation, in MSB broth with 15 % glycerol concentration. We recommend combining equal volumes of overnight cultures in MSB broth and 30 % sterile glycerol.

8. This method is based on O'Callagham and Charbit [68]. Note that the settings are different for 1 and 2 mm cuvettes and for the strain. Using 2 mm cuvettes we use 2.5 kV, 1000 Ω, and 25 µF for the *Salmonella* strain YS8211 and 2.5 kV, 400 Ω, and 25 µF for suppressed strains and the ATCC wild type strain 14028. Many labs generate large numbers of competent cells using 250 ml centrifuge bottles and rotors such as the Sorvall GSA. However, large rotors take significant time to stop, and larger pellets are difficult to resuspend homogeneously. Given the number of centrifuge runs in this protocol, large scale preparation takes considerable time. Since only a few of electro-competent cells are needed in this protocol, the long spin and stopping times and lengthy resuspension times are replaced with 1 min centrifugations and 30 s. resuspensions, generating a significantly more rapid protocol for the generation of electro-competent cells.

9. When the culture is nearing OD_{600} 0.6, it will be in log phase and growing extremely fast. The spectrophotometer should be in proximity to the bacterial-shaking incubator in order to minimize the time between taking a subsample and its spectrophotometric reading. The reading should be recorded immediately, and if the culture has reached the desired OD_{600}, the shaker flask should be immediately placed on ice with gentle swirling to rapidly cool it down. Note that not all of the bacterial culture is used. Standardization of ~1:100 dilution to start

the culture facilitates uniformity within a lab generating different amounts of competent cells at different times.

10. Autoclaving liquids at 15 lbs for 15 min is the simplest and least expensive method for sterilizing glycerol-water pressure solutions. Alternatively, solutions may be sterilized using a 0.22 μm vacuum filtration system.

11. Gently pipette the liquid to the bottom of the cuvette, being careful to avoid introduction of bubbles which can result in arcing of the electric current and not successfully electroporating the cells.

12. The time constant should generally be between 4 and 7 ms when using 1 mm cuvettes, and between 6 and 9 when using 2 mm cuvettes. Times outside of that range, especially shorter times are usually ineffective and often indicate the presence of conductive ions which the extensive water–glycerol washes are meant to eliminate.

13. Phosphate-buffered saline (PBS) should not be used for the strain YS8211 which is sensitive to PBS.

14. pNK2883 carries a Tn*10* transposon that only confers tet_{20}^{R} after it integrates into the chromosome. The transposase for the Tn*10* is under control of an IPTG-inducible promoter.

15. *Salmonella* serovar Typhimurium LT2 has ~4500 annotated genes [69]; therefore, a minimum of 22,500 colonies must be plated for five-fold coverage of the genome. To pick the best dilution for plating the Tn*10* library, select a dilution that will yield well-separated colonies (calculation of CFU/ml by doing a dilution series or by diluting the culture to a particular OD of known CFU/ml is required to optimize this procedure). You will also need additional plates containing at least 1000 colonies for analysis of the transposon library (see next section). These additional plates will serve as master plates—therefore, it is critical that the colonies are well-separated.

16. A random Tn*10* library will contain auxotrophic mutants in various nucleotide or amino-acid biosynthetic pathways.

17. It is critical to resuspend the cells directly from the agar plates rather than growing them in liquid because slow-growing colonies are not directly competing with other colonies on a well-separated spread plate. In a liquid culture, cells with faster doubling times will take over the culture.

18. The P22-sensitive bacterial culture can be kept at 4 °C for weeks.

19. One Tn*10* library can be used to link Tn*10*s in many different suppressor strains by creating one phage P22 Tn*10* transducing library.

20. Do not use polystyrene tubes, which can be easily dissolved by chloroform. Use of glass tubes is recommended.

21. For ATCC 14028, a 0.400 OD_{600} indicates $\sim 2.0 \times 10^8$ CFU/ml.

22. Do not use MSB agar, because the Mg^{2+} and Ca^{2+} in MSB agar promote phage contamination.

23. The soft agar helps to protect transductants from virulent phage. 0.5 % soft agar results in larger phage plaques; 0.6 % soft agar will result in smaller plaques. Also note that the alizarin yellow dye in green plates cannot be used for testing for *Salmonella* infected with phage, as *msbB Salmonella* do not grow on green agar plates.

24. Co-transduction frequency reflects the frequency of the transposon (Tn*10*) associated with the suppressor gene (co-transduction). A transposon near the suppressor gene will only sometimes bring the suppressor gene along with it. The closer the transposon and the suppressor mutation, the more frequently they will be co-transduced. The co-transduction frequency reflects to the number (e.g., 16 out of 30) of tet^R transductants with restored EGTA sensitivity (that now have a wild-type copy of the suppressor gene; the other 14 tet^R transductants would still be $EGTA^R$). Use the following equation to estimate the distance (in Kb) between the transposon and the suppressor mutation: co-transduction frequency = (1−(distance between 2 markers in Kb)/(length of transducing particle genome)^3 [70]. (The P22 genome is 41.7 Kb.) In this case, the co-transduction frequency is 0.53 (16/30) and the distance between the transposon and suppressor mutation is 7.95 Kb.

25. In experiments to determine the co-transduction frequency, two types of strains will be created: (1) those linking the transposon to the wild-type allele and (2) others linking the transposon to the mutant allele of the suppressor gene. Both are of value and can be used to transduce either the wild-type or the mutant allele of the suppressor gene into a new genetic background.

26. Use new TAE running buffer in a clean gel box to reduce the chance of DNA cross-contamination.

27. Use long wavelength UV (e.g., 365 nm) and keep the gel on the its tray to prevent molecular contamination from the UV-source surface.

28. Set up a control ligation without insert. This will detect either an uncut or re-ligated vector.

29. Sensitivity of *msbB* mutants to CO_2 was first observed during the human clinical trial at the National Cancer Institute [21]. It was noted that VNP20009 grew best at 37 °C without

added CO_2 after a standard CO_2 tissue culture chamber was used for incubation of the serial dilutions of the bacteria from the frozen vials that were produced for the clinical trial. In the protocol that we describe, a standard air + CO_2 chamber can be used with CO_2 at 5 % to obtain the desired effect.

30. It is extremely important that the library be plated in a manner such that all the colonies are evenly spaced on all of the plates in order to minimize over representation of certain clones. Both faster-growing and slower-growing clones can be expected. Plating the colonies at a relatively high density resulting in smaller colonies the size of a pin head is generally beneficial in this regard.

31. There should be about 10,000 or greater colonies per 150 mm plate, which achieves 5× or greater coverage of the genome coding sequences, assuming random insertion of the transposons.

32. A library harvested as described will typically have a density of 1×10^{11} CFU/ml. Since the complexity of the library may be 30,000 clones (representing 5× or greater coverage), a single microliter of the library may contain more than 1000-fold coverage of the library.

33. A typical result will show a two-log or greater decrease in the plating efficiency of the library on the first round of selection. Later rounds and individually-selected clones may show improvements of approximately two orders of magnitude.

34. Due to the presence spontaneous suppressors among individuals of the transposon-insertion library where the clones are both kanamycin resistant and CO_2 resistant, but where CO_2 resistance is not due to the transposon, linkage of the transposon and CO_2 resistance among the clones found on the first round of selection is not as likely as in subsequent rounds of purification, hence we conduct an enrichment as described in Sub-heading 3.3.4.

35. LB-0 works better than MSB since there is no calcium or magnesium to interfere with the EDTA.

36. Washes are necessary to get rid of any virulent wild-type phage that might infect the bacteria and cause lysis. Since VNP20009 (YS1646) is somewhat sensitive to 10 mM EGTA this could result in selection for additional suppressor mutations. Therefore it is necessary to use lower EGTA amounts and take off as much supernatant as possible in each wash to remove the greatest amount of phage possible.

37. We recommend testing multiple strains of *Salmonella* following the design and derivation of new strains. While the strains such as VNP20009 that we previously generated have shown a

high degree of genetic stability [71], not all strains derived independently show the same antitumor activity. For example, the strain VNP20008 which was derived using the same procedure to derive VNP20009, only showed 44 % tumor inhibition in the B16F10 tumor model, whereas VNP20009 typically exhibited greater than 90 % inhibition (unpublished data).

Acknowledgments

This work was supported by start-up funds from the California State University, Northridge College of Mathematics and Science (for DB). KBL, JP, and DB express their admiration for the late Helen Coley Nauts (1907–2001) and appreciation for her meeting with them in April 2000 to discuss the work of her late father William B. Coley. We also thank the anonymous reviewers for their helpful comments.

References

1. Hall SS (1997) A commotion in the blood: Life, death, and the immune system. Henry Holt, New York

2. Nauts HC, Swift WE, Coley BL (1946) The treatment of malignant tumors by bacterial toxins as developed by the late William B. Coley, MD, reviewed in the light of modern research. Cancer Res 6:205–216

3. Coley WB (1891) Contribution to the knowledge of sarcoma. Ann Surg 14:199–220

4. Fehleisen F (1883) Die etiologie des erysipels. Berlin. (as cited by Coley in Ref. 3)

5. Parker RC, Plummer HC, Siebenmann CO, Chapman MG (1947) Effect of histolyticus infection and toxin on transplantable mouse tumors. Proc Soc Exp Biol Med 66:461–467

6. Möse JR, Möse G (1964) Oncolysis by clostridia. I. Activity of *Clostridium butyricum* (M-55) and other nonpathogenic clostridia against the Ehrlich carcinoma. Cancer Res 24:212–216

7. Carey RW, Holland JF, Whang HY, Neter E, Bryant B (1967) Clostridial oncolysis in man. Eur J Cancer 3:37–46

8. Fox ME, Lemmon M, Mauchline ML, Davis TO, Giaccia AJ, Minton NP, Brown JM (1996) Anaerobic bacteria as a delivery system for cancer gene therapy: In vitro activation of 5-fluorocytosine by genetically engineered clostridia. Gene Ther 3:173–178

9. Dang LH, Bettegowda C, Huso DL, Kinzler KW, Vogelstein B (2001) Combination bacteriolytic therapy for the treatment of experimental tumors. Proc Natl Acad Sci U S A 98:15155–15160

10. Dolgin E (2011) From spinach scare to cancer care. Nat Med 17:273–275

11. Forbes NS (2010) Engineering the perfect (bacterial) cancer therapy. Nat Rev Cancer 10:785–794

12. Bermudes D, Low KB, Pawelek JM (2000) Tumor-targeted *Salmonella*. Highly selective delivery vectors. Adv Exp Med Biol 465:57–63

13. Bermudes D, Low KB, Pawelek J (2000) Tumor-targeted *Salmonella*: Strain development and expression of the HSV TK effector gene. In: Walther W, Stein U (eds) Gene therapy: methods and protocols, vol 35. Humana, Totowa, NJ, pp 419–436

14. Darveau R (1999) Infection, inflammation and cancer. Nat Biotechnol 17:19

15. Low KB, Ittensohn M, Le T, Platt J, Sodi S, Amoss M, Ash O, Carmichael E, Chakraborty A, Fisher J, Lin SL, Luo X, Miller SI, Zheng Limou King I, Pawelek JM, Bermudes D (1999) Lipid A mutant *Salmonella* with suppressed virulence and TNFα induction retain tumor-targeting *in vivo*. Nat Biotechnol 17:37–41

16. Pawelek JM, Low KB, Bermudes D (1997) Tumor-targeted *Salmonella* as a novel anticancer vector. Cancer Res 57:4537–4544

17. Pawelek JM, Low KB, Bermudes D (2003) Bacteria as tumour-targeting vectors. Lancet Oncol 4:548–556

18. ClinicalTrials.gov. Identifier: NCT01118819, Safety study of *Clostridium novyi*-NT spores to treat patients with solid tumors that have not responded to standard therapies

19. ClinicalTrials.gov. Identifier: NCT01598792, Safety study of recombinant *Listeria monocytogenes* (Lm) based vaccine virus vaccine to treat oropharyngeal Cancer (REALISTIC)

20. ClinicalTrials.gov. Identifier: NCT01675765, CRS-207 Cancer vaccine in combination with chemotherapy as front-line treatment for malignant pleural mesothelioma

21. Toso JF, Gill VJ, Hwu P, Marincola FM, Restifo NP, Schwartzentruber DJ, Sherry RM, Topalian SL, Yang JC, Stock F, Freezer LJ, Morton KE, Seipp C, Haworth L, Mavroukakis S, White D, MacDonald S, Mao J, Sznol M, Rosenberg SA (2002) Phase I study of the intravenous administration of attenuated *Salmonella* typhimurium to patients with metastatic melanoma. J Clin Oncol 20:142–152

22. Nemunaitis J, Cunningham C, Senzer N, Kuhn J, Cramm J, Litz C, Cavagnolo R, Cahill A, Clairmont C, Sznol M (2003) Pilot trial of genetically modified, attenuated *Salmonella* expressing the *E. coli* cytosine deaminase gene in refractory cancer patients. Cancer Gene Ther 10:737–744

23. ClinicalTrials.gov. Identifier: NCT00004988, Treatment of patients with cancer with genetically modified *Salmonella typhimurium* bacteria

24. Zhao M, Yang M, Li X-M, Jiang P, Li S, Xu M, Hoffman RM (2005) Tumor-targeting bacterial therapy with amino acid auxotrophs of GFP-expressing *Salmonella typhimurium*. Proc Natl Acad Sci U S A 102:755–760

25. Zhao M, Yang M, Ma H, Li X, Tan X, Li S, Yang Z, Hoffman RM (2006) Targeted therapy with a *Salmonella typhimurium* leucine-arginine auxotroph cures orthotopic human breast tumors in nude mice. Cancer Res 66:7647–7652

26. Zhao M, Geller J, Ma H, Yang M, Penman S, Hoffman RM (2007) Monotherapy with a tumor-targeting mutant of *Salmonella typhimurium* cures orthotopic metastatic mouse models of human prostate cancer. Proc Natl Acad Sci U S A 104:10170–10174

27. Hiroshima Y, Zhao M, Zhang Y, Maawy A, Hassanein MK, Uehara F, Miwa S, Yano S, Momiyama M, Suetsugu A, Chishima T, Tanaka K, Bouvet M, Endo I, Hoffman RM (2013) Comparison of efficacy of *Salmonella typhimurium* A1-R and chemotherapy on stem-like and non-stem human pancreatic cancer cells. Cell Cycle 12:2774–2780

28. ClinicalTrials.gov. Identifier: NCT01099631, IL-2 expressing, attenuated *Salmonella typhimurium* in unresectable hepatic spread

29. Low KB, Ittensohn M, Luo X, Zheng L-M, King I, Pawelek JM, Bermudes D (2004) Construction of VNP20009, a novel, genetically stable antibiotic sensitive strain of tumor-targeting *Salmonella* for parenteral administration in humans. Methods Mol Med 90:47–60

30. Murray SR, Bermudes D, de Felipe KS, Low KB (2001) Extragenic suppressors of growth defects in *msbB Salmonella*. J Bacteriol 183:5554–5561

31. Murray SR, Suwwan de Felipe K, Obuchowski PL, Pike J, Bermudes D, Low KB (2004) Hot spot for a large deletion in the 18–19 Cs region confers a multiple phenotype in *Salmonella enterica* serovar Typhimurium strain ATCC 14028. J Bacteriol 186:8516–8523

32. Murray SR, Ernst RK, Bermudes D, Miller SI, Low KB (2007) PmrA(Con) confers *pmrHFIJKL*-dependent EGTA and polymyxin resistance on *msbB Salmonella* by decorating Lipid A with phosphoethanolamine. J Bacteriol 189:5161–5169

33. Karsten V, Murray SR, Pike J, Troy K, Ittensohn M, Kondradzhyan M, Low KB, Bermudes D (2009) *msbB* deletion confers acute sensitivity to CO_2 in *Salmonella enterica* serovar Typhimurium that can be suppressed by a loss-of-function mutation in zwf. BMC Microbiol 189:170. doi:10.1186/1471-2180-9-170.33

34. Karow M, Georgopoulos C (1992) Isolation and characterization of the *Escherichia coli msbB* gene, a multicopy suppressor of null mutations in the high-temperature requirement gene *htrB*. J Bacteriol 174:702–710

35. Engel H, Smink AJ, van Wijngaarden L, Keck W (1992) Murine-metabolizing enzymes from *Escherichia coli*: existence of a second lytic transglycosylase. J Bacteriol 174:6394–6403

36. Kahn SA, Everest P, Servos S, Foxwell N, Zahringer U, Brade H, Rietschel ET, Dougan G, Charles IG, Maskell D (1998) A lethal role for lipid a in *Salmonella* infections. Mol Microbiol 29:571–579

37. Carty S, Sreekumar K, Raetz C (1999) Effect of cold shock on lipid A biosynthesis in *Escherichia coli*. J Biol Chem 274:9677–9685

38. Baker SJ, Markowitz S, Fearon ER, Willson JK, Vogelstein B (1990) Suppression of human colorectal carcinoma cell growth by wild-type p53. Science 249:912–915

39. Beadle GW, Ephrussi B (1936) Development of eye colors in *Drosophila*: transplantation experiments with suppressor of vermilion. Proc Natl Acad Sci U S A 22:536–540

40. Crick F, Barnett L, Brenner S, Watts-Tobin JR (1961) General nature of the genetic code for proteins. Nature 192:1227–1232

41. Bossi L, Roth JR (1981) Four-base codons ACCA, ACCU and ACCC are recognized by the frameshift suppressor *sufJ*. Cell 24: 489–496

42. Ruiz N, Falcone B, Kahne D, Silhavy TJ (2005) Chemical conditionality: a genetic strategy to probe organelle assembly. Cell 121:307–317

43. Ruiz N, Kahne D, Silhavy TJ (2006) Advances in understanding bacterial outer-membrane biogenesis. Nat Rev Microbiol 4:57–66

44. Silhavy TJ, Kahane D, Walker S (2010) The bacterial cell envelope. In: Shapiro L, Losick R (eds) Cell Biology of Bacteria. Cold Spring Harbor Laboratory Press, Plainview, NY, pp 79–94

45. Wu T, Malinverni J, Ruiz N, Kim S, Silhavy TJ, Kahne D (2005) Identification of a multi-component complex required for outer membrane biogenesis. Cell 121:235–245

46. Beckwith J (2009) Genetic suppressors and recovery of repressed biochemical memory. J Biol Chem 284:12585–12592

47. Hartman PE, Roth JR (1973) Mechanisms of suppression. Adv Genet 17:1–105

48. Michels CA (2002) Suppression analysis. Chapter 8, In: CA Michels (Eds) Genetic techniques for biological research: A case study approach. Wiley and Sons. pp. 91–98. doi: 10.1002/0470846623

49. Prelich G (1999) Suppression mechanisms: themes and variations. Trends Genet 15:261–266

50. Okuda S, Tokuda H (2011) Lipoprotein sorting in bacteria. Annu Rev Microbiol 65: 239–259

51. Raivio TL, Silhavy TJ (2001) Periplasmic stress and ECF sigma factors. Annu Rev Microbiol 55:591–624

52. Ruiz N, Silhavy TJ (2005) Sensing external stress: watchdogs of the *Escherichia coli* cell envelope. Curr Opin Microbiol 8:122–126

53. De Las Penas A, Connolly L, Gross CA (1997) Sigma[E] is an essential sigma factor in *Escherichia coli*. J Bacteriol 179:6862–6864

54. Alba BM, Gross CA (2004) Regulation of the *Escherichia coli* sigma-dependent envelope stress response. Mol Microbiol 52:613–619

55. Button JE, Silhavy TJ, Ruiz N (2007) A suppressor of cell death caused by the loss of sigma[E] downregulates extracytoplasmic stress responses and outer membrane vesicle production in *Escherichia coli*. J Bacteriol 189:1523–1530

56. Hayden JD, Ades SE (2008) The extracytoplasmic stress factor, σ[E], is required to maintain cell envelope integrity in *Escherichia coli*. PLoS One 3(2), e1573. doi:10.1371/journal.pone.0001573

57. Rowley G, Spector M, Kormanec J, Roberts M (2006) Pushing the envelope: extracytoplasmic stress responses in bacterial pathogens. Nat Rev Microbiol 4:383–394

58. Paradis-Bleau C, Markovski M, Uehara T, Lupoli TJ, Walker S, Kahne DE, Bernhardt TG (2010) Lipoprotein cofactors located in the outer membrane activate bacterial cell wall polymerases. Cell 143:1110–112026

59. Typas A, Banzhaf M, van Saparoea B, Verheul J, Bilboy J, Nichols RJ, Zietek M, Beilharz K, Kannenberg K, von Rechenberg M, Breukink E, den Blaauwen T, Gross CA, Vollmer W (2010) Regulation of peptidoglycan synthesis by outer-membrane proteins. Cell 143: 1097–1109

60. Qi S-Y, Sukupolvi S, O'Connor CD (1991) Outer membrane permeability of *Escherichia coli* K12: Isolation, cloning and mapping of suppressors of a defined antibiotic-hypersensitive mutant. Mol Gen Genet 229:421–427

61. Tsai SP, Hartin RJ, Ryu J-I (1989) Transformation in restriction-deficient *Salmonella typhimurium* LT2. J Gen Microbiol 135:2561–2567

62. Kleckner N, Bender J, Gottesman S (1991) Uses of transposons with emphasis on the Tn*10*. Methods Enzymol 204:139–180

63. Miller JH (1992) A short course in bacterial genetics. Cold Spring Harbor Laboratory Press, Plainview, NY

64. Sambrook J, Fritsch EF, Maniatis T (1989) Molecular cloning: a laboratory manual. Cold Spring Harbor Laboratory Press, Plainview, NY

65. Marmur J (1961) A procedure for the isolation of deoxyribonucleic acid from microorganism. J Mol Biol 3:208–21848

66. Kolodkin AL, Capage MA, Golub EI, Low KB (1983) F sex factor of *Escherichia coli* K-12 codes for a single-stranded DNA binding protein. Proc Natl Acad Sci U S A 80: 4422–4426

67. Siebert PD, Chenchik A, Kellogg DE, Lukyanov KA, Lukyanov SA (1995) An improved PCR method for walking in uncloned genomic DNA. Nucleic Acids Res 23:1087–1088

68. O'Callaghan D, Charbit A (1990) High efficiency transformation of *Salmonella typhimurium* and *Salmonella typhi* by electroporation. Mol Gen Genet 223:156–158

69. McClelland M, Sanderson KE, Spieth J, Clifton SW, Latreille P, Courtney L, Porwollik S, Ali J, Dante M, Du F, Hou S, Layman D, Leonard S, Nguyen C, Scott K, Holmes A,

Grewal N, Mulvaney E, Ryan E, Sun H, Florea L, Miller W, Stoneking T, Nhan M, Waterston RK (2001) Complete genome sequence of Salmonella enterica serovar Typhimurium LT2. Nature 413:852–856

70. Wu TT (1966) A model for three-point analysis of random generalized transduction. Genetics 54:405–410

71. Clairmont C, Lee KC, Pike J, Ittensohn M, Low KB, Pawelek J, Bermudes D, Brecher SM, Margitich D, Turnier J, Li Z, Luo X, King I, Zheng L-M (2000) Biodistribution and genetic stability of the novel antitumor agent VNP20009, a genetically modified strain of *Salmonella typhimurium*. J Infect Dis 181:1996–2002

Chapter 11

Determination of Plasmid Segregational Stability in a Growing Bacterial Population

M. Gabriela Kramer

Abstract

Bacterial plasmids are extensively used as cloning vectors for a number of genes for academic and commercial purposes. Moreover, attenuated bacteria carrying recombinant plasmids expressing genes with anti-tumor activity have shown promising therapeutic results in animal models of cancer. Equitable plasmid distribution between daughter cells during cell division, i.e., plasmid segregational stability, depends on many factors, including the plasmid copy number, its replication mechanism, the levels of recombinant gene expression, the type of bacterial host, and the metabolic burden associated with all these factors. Plasmid vectors usually code for antibiotic-resistant functions, and, in order to enrich the culture with bacteria containing plasmids, antibiotic selective pressure is commonly used to eliminate plasmid-free segregants from the growing population. However, administration of antibiotics can be inconvenient for many industrial and therapeutic applications. Extensive ongoing research is being carried out to develop stably-inherited plasmid vectors. Here, I present an easy and precise method for determining the kinetics of plasmid loss or maintenance for every ten generations of bacterial growth in culture.

Key words Plasmid, Stability, Cell division, Bacterial population

1 Introduction

Plasmids are extra-chromosomal genetic elements that replicate and segregate independently of the bacterial chromosome, although these functions depend to a high extent on the host's enzymes [1, 2]. In some cases, especially naturally-occurring low-copy-number plasmids, carry active partitioning functions that ensure that each daughter cell receives a plasmid copy at cell division [3, 4]. They are also toxin-antitoxin stability systems, based on the selective killing of plasmid-free segregants [4, 5]. For high-copy-number plasmids, intra-molecular resolution of dimer formation during replication and/or random plasmid distribution to daughter cells generally operates in the absence of selective pressure [6]. In addition, plasmid stability depends on it's type of replication mechanisms, the bacterial host, and functional cross talk between them aimed to balance the metabolic burden imposed by

Robert M. Hoffman (ed.), *Bacterial Therapy of Cancer: Methods and Protocols*, Methods in Molecular Biology, vol. 1409, DOI 10.1007/978-1-4939-3515-4_11, © Springer Science+Business Media New York 2016

plasmids [7–10]. Most commercially-available plasmid vectors used for recombinant gene expression are present in high copy number and contain antibiotic-resistance genes to eliminate plasmid-free bacteria from a growing population in case they behave unstably. In these cases, plasmid stability can be also affected by factors such as the nature of the recombinant gene and it's expression levels [11]. However, the use of antibiotics to produce proteins at an industrial level is currently becoming more restricted owing to the possibility of contamination of the final product. In addition, the use of antibiotics to select bacteria containing plasmids expressing anti-tumor or antigenic genes might be inconvenient for cancer therapy or vaccination [11–14]. Therefore, the development of expression plasmids that can be stably maintained in a desired bacterial host in the absence of antibiotics, as well as a precise plasmid stability test that can be easily applied for comparative studies has both industrial and therapeutic relevance.

As a model system, I will describe here the stability test of a hypothetical high-copy-number plasmid vector (pAmp) carrying an ampicillin (Amp)-resistance gene in a facultative anaerobic Gram (–) Enterobacteriaceae such as *Escherichia coli* (*E. coli*). Such a method has been used to determine the segregation stability of various natural and constructed plasmids in a number of Gram (–) and Gram (+) bacteria [7, 15, 16]. This method can be applied to any bacterial plasmid that encodes an antibiotic-resistance gene, regardless its size and copy number. The composition of the culture media, temperature and time of incubation, shaking conditions, oxygen supply, type and concentration of selective agent, as well as biosafety regulations needs to be adapted for the particular bacteria-plasmid system that is being used. Moreover, as long as the selective conditions can be reproduced in culture, this method can be adjusted to any other kind of selective advantage conferred by plasmids to their bacterial host, such as the resistance to metal ions or the supply of an enzyme for an metabolic function.

2 Materials (*See* Note 1)

1. Luria-Bertani (LB) broth [17, 18] (*see* **Note 2**).
2. LB-agar plates (*see* **Notes 3–7**).
3. Amp stock solutions (*see* **Notes 8** and **9**).
4. Glycerol stock solution (*see* **Note 10**).

3 Methods

The present method is described for analyzing the segregational stability of pAmp in *E. coli* at its exponential (mid-log) growth phase. It is based on the quantification of the percentage of Amp-resistant bacteria successively measured every 10 generations during 50 generations of cell division. This procedure allows the determination of the kinetics of plasmid loss in case the plasmid is unstable and may take several days according to the results for the initial generations. If plasmids are very unstable, then, only 10–30 generation analysis may be required; however, long-term assays may be necessary for plasmids with low loss rates.

3.1 Collection of E. coli-pAmp Culture Samples Every Ten Growing Generations

1. To obtain Generation 0 (G0), prepare a 3 ml overnight (O/N, 12–18 h) culture of E. coli-pAmp in liquid LB medium containing 100 μg/ml Amp (see **Note 11**). If possible, start from a single colony obtained from a streaked Amp-LB-agar plate (see **Note 12**). Grow the culture at 37 °C + shaker at 200–250 rpm.

2. Dilute the O/N culture 1/100 in fresh LB media with Amp and let it grow in the same conditions as described above. Measure the optical density (OD) at 600 nm in a spectrophotometer every 20–30 min (the aliquot volume for OD measurement will depend on the equipment used, ranging from 1 μl to 1 ml) (see **Note 13**). While the aliquot is being measured, keep the culture incubated on ice to stop bacterial growth.

3. When cultures reach $OD_{600} = 0.5$ (mid-log phase) (see **Note 14**), make two 16–17 % glycerol stocks (600 μl of culture + 300 μl glycerol [50 %]) in sterile screw-cap cryo-tubes (see **Note 15**). Mix well by vortexing, incubate 5 min on ice, and store both tubes at –80 °C (see **Note 16**).

4. Keep the rest of the culture incubated on ice for performing dilutions and bacteria plating the same day (go to Sub-heading 3.2) (see **Note 17**). G0 is meant to be the starting point, a mid-log phase culture where 100 % of bacteria contain the plasmid.

5. To obtain Generation 10 (G10), the next day (see **Note 18**), completely thaw one of the G0 frozen glycerol stocks by incubating the cryotube on ice for about 30 min. Mix well with a vortex.

6. Inoculate a $1/1024^{(*)(**)}$ dilution of the thawed G0 in fresh LB media without antibiotic (see **Note 13**). Measure the OD until the culture reaches $OD_{600} = 0.5$. Then proceed as for G0 and make two 16–17 % glycerol stocks (see above). Keep the rest of the culture incubated on ice for performing bacteria plating (go to Sub-heading 3.2) (see **Note 17**).

   $^{(*)}$ If the bacterial population obtained in G0 is diluted 1/1024 in LB media and cultured again until it reaches $OD_{600} = 0.5$, it would undergo ten divisions. This reasoning is derived from the following equation, which is applicable to any kind of population governed by exponential growth dynamics:

$$N_2 = N_1 \times 2^G$$

   In the present case, N_1 is the number of starting bacteria required to reach N_2 (number of bacteria at $OD_{600} = 0.5$) after several generations (G) of exponential growth. If the number of generations is 10, then

$$N_2 = N_1 \times 2^{10} = N_1 \times 1024$$
$$N_1 = N_2 \times 1/1024.$$

Therefore, by inoculating $1/1024$ of G0 at $OD_{600} = 0.5$ (100 % bacteria containing plasmid) in LB medium without antibiotic and letting it grow up to $OD_{600} = 0.5$, we would have again N_2 bacteria that went through ten generations of cell division, obtaining G10 (here, the percentage of bacteria containing plasmid would depend on its segregational stability, since no Amp was added).

$^{(**)}$ Frozen 16–17 % glycerol stocks are comprised of $2/3$ bacteria culture (600 µl) + $1/3$ glycerol 50 % (300 µl); therefore, a correction factor of 1.5 should be added to the inoculum volume, i.e., for each 1022.5 µl of fresh LB media, add 1.5 µl of the thawed glycerol stock in order to obtain an exact $1/1024$ dilution of the bacteria culture.

7. To obtain Generation 20 (G20), the following day, completely thaw one of the G10 frozen glycerol stocks as indicated above and dilute it $1/1024^{(**)}$ in fresh LB medium without antibiotic. Measure the OD of the growing culture at 600 nm. When the culture reaches $OD_{600} = 0.5$, proceed as for G0 and G10.

8. To obtain Generation 30 (G30), G40, and G50, make subsequent $1/1024^{(**)}$ dilutions of G20-, G30-, and G40-thawed cultures in LB medium without selective pressure and let it grow until $OD_{600} = 0.5$ (*see* **Note 18**).

9. In all cases, keep part of the grown culture incubated on ice for performing suitable dilutions and bacteria plating the same day (*see* Sub-heading 3.2) (*see* **Note 17**).

3.2 Quantification of Bacteria Containing pAmp in G0–G50 Cultures

The percentage of bacteria containing plasmid (B + P) is calculated by plating suitable diluted samples of G0–G50 populations at $OD_{600} = 0.5$ in LB-agar and in Amp-LB-agar plates. The addition of Amp to the plate allows for the selection of only those bacteria carrying pAmp. G0 cultures were grown with Amp; therefore, it is expected that (B + P) = 100 %. G10–G50 cultures were grown without Amp; therefore, if pAmp is segregationally stable, then (B + P) is expected to continue being 100 %. However, if pAmp is unstable, this percentage will decrease during the next generations according it's particular kinetics of plasmid loss.

1. To confirm 100 % (B + P) at G0, make serial $1/10$ dilutions in PBS ($1\times$) of the G0 culture at $OD_{600} = 0.5$, obtained as described in Sub-heading 3.1, **steps 1–4** (*see* **Note 19**).

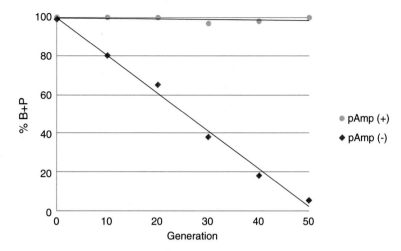

Fig. 1 Example of the percentage (%) of bacteria containing plasmid (B + P) that could be obtained in case the hypothetical pAmp plasmid is stable (+) or unstable (−) in the selected bacterial host population during 50 growth generations

2. Plate 20–100 μl of the suitable dilution/s in order to obtain 50–200 colony-forming units (CFU)/plate with or without Amp (*see* **Notes 19–21**). Let plates dry in a sterile atmosphere, close the lids, invert the plates, and incubate them O/N at 37 °C.

3. Calculate the CFU/ml in both LB-agar and Amp-LB-agar plates (*see* **Notes 20**). Calculate the percentage (%) of bacteria containing plasmid (B + P) using the following equation:

$$\% \ (B+P) = (CFU/ml \ in \ Amp\text{-}LB\text{-}agar \ / \ CFU/ml \ in \ LB\text{-}agar) \times 100$$

4. To calculate the % (B + P) for G10, make serial 1/10 dilutions in PBS (1×) of the G10 culture at $OD_{600} = 0.5$ obtained as described in Sub-heading 3.1, **steps 5–6** (*see* **Note 19**). Plate 20–100 μl of the *estimated* dilutions (*see* **Note 21**) in LB-agar and Amp-LB-agar and proceed as above.

5. To calculate the % (B + P) for G20, G30, G40, and G50, make serial dilutions of the G20, G30, G40, and G50 cultures ($OD_{600} = 0.5$) obtained as described in Subheading 3.1, **steps 7–9**, and proceed as for G0 and G10.

Figure 1 describes a putative result that could be expected in case pAmp is stable (+) or unstable (−) in *E. coli*. The slope of the curve would give complementary information if comparing the kinetics of loss of different unstable plasmids.

4   Notes

1. All culture media and working stock solutions must be sterilized by autoclaving or filtration through 0.2 µm pores. LB-agar plate preparation and manipulation of bacteria samples (cultures and plating) require confinement to a sterile working area in the laboratory. A Class II HEPA-filtered air cabinet would be most appropriate. If such a cabinet is not available, select an area of the laboratory that is far away from air turbulences and install a laboratory Bunsen burner and keep the flame (blue) on during the whole manipulation period. Always wipe the bench surface, tube racks, and micropipettes with 70 % ethanol before starting. The ethanol bottle should be at a safety distance away from burner. Never leave the burner on unattended to avoid fire accidents. Opening of bacteria-containing tubes, plating, and pipetting should be carefully done in order to reduce the risk of bacterial aerosol formation and cross-contamination when working with more than one culture. Keep an ice bucket next to the working area for bacteria incubation. Diligently follow biological waste-disposal regulations.

2. LB preparation: Luria-Bertani (LB) broth [17, 18] is a nutrient-rich medium widely used for the growth of bacteria. To prepare 500 ml of LB, dissolve 5 g NaCl, 5 g tryptone, and 2.5 g yeast extract in 450 ml de-ionized water (dH$_2$O) in an autoclave-resistant flask. Adjust the pH of the solution to 7.0 with NaOH and bring the volume up to 500 ml with dH$_2$O. Autoclave liquids for 20 min. Cool down at room temperature. LB medium can be also purchased as sterile liquid and premixed powder.

3. LB-agar preparation: To prepare 500 ml sufficient for approximately 25 LB-agar plates, mix 5 g NaCl, 5 g tryptone, 2.5 g yeast extract, 7.5 g agar, and dH$_2$O to 500 ml (*see* **Note 4**). Autoclave liquid for 20 min. If used in the same day, allow the agar solution to cool down to 50 °C by placing the flask in a 50 °C oven or water bath. Otherwise, let LB-agar solidify at room temperature and melt it when needed (*see* **Note 5**). To prepare LB-agar plates with antibiotic (Amp-LB-agar), add 100 µg/ml Amp to the 50 °C liquid LB-agar before poring it into the Petri dish (*see* **Note 6**). Pour 20–25 ml per 10 cm polystyrene Petri dish. Place the lids off the plates to avoid vapor condensation on the lid and allow the LB-agar to cool until solidified (30–60 min). Then place lids on, invert the plates, and store in plastic bags or sealed with Parafilm (to prevent dehydration) at 4 °C (*see* **Note 7**). LB-agar can be also purchased from commercial sources.

4. If premixed LB-agar powder is available, use the suggested amount instead of the indicated reagents.

5. Solid LB-agar can be stored in autoclaved flasks for several months at room temperature. To melt it again, incubate the flask in a boiling water bath until no clumps are seen and/or melt it using a microwave. Loosen the cap before putting the flask in the microwave and let it stay for several minutes before taking it out to prevent the boiling liquid from coming out from the flask.

6. Make sure the temperature of the LB-agar is approximately 50 °C. If the solution is too warm, it may degrade the antibiotic or damage the Petri plates. If the solution is too cool, it may solidify before the plates are poured.

7. LB-agar plates can be stored at 4 °C in a closed plastic bag or sealed with Parafilm for 1–2 months. Amp-LB-agar plates may only last for several weeks at 4 °C. It is advised that long-term stored antibiotic plates are tested with the right controls before using.

8. Antibiotic preparation: Amp stock solutions (100 mg/ml, 1000×) can be prepared in sterile dH_2O and sterilized by 0.2 μm pore filtration (see **Note 9**). Store at –20 °C in small aliquots and allow no more than ten freezing-thawing cycles.

9. Never autoclave antibiotics; they can be inactivated with high temperature. Amp can be also prepared in 70 % ethanol if used in a short-time period. There are two advantages to this method: the solution is liquid at –20 °C and it is self sterilizing. But the disadvantage is that the solution is unstable, since ethanol is a weak catalyst of b-lactam ring disruption.

10. Glycerol solution: Glycerol stock solution at 50 % is prepared by diluting one volume of 100 % glycerol in a same volume of dH_2O or PBS (1×) (phosphate-buffered saline). Autoclave and store at room temperature. The addition of glycerol stabilizes the frozen bacteria, preventing damage to the cell membranes and keeping the cells alive. Glycerol stocks of bacteria (15–25 %) can be stored at –80 °C for many years; however, bacteria viability decreases with repeated freezing-thawing cycles.

11. Plasmid copy number can vary, depending on the bacterial host. A selective medium containing 100 μg/ml Amp is recommended for high-copy-number plasmids (≥100) carrying the Amp-resistant gene; if plasmid copy number is lower, it would be preferable to use 50 μg/ml Amp.

12. Using a sterile toothpick or pipette tip, touch the bacteria colony growing in the Amp-LB-agar plate and disperse the bacteria in fresh LB + Amp culture medium. All bacteria liquid cultures are grown at 37 °C + shaker at 200–250 rpm.

13. The culture volume will depend on the type of spectrophotometer used to measure OD_{600} (i.e., if the sample needs to be 0.5 ml, one may predict about 5–7 measurements, and then a 6 ml culture may be enough).

14. The OD for mid-log phase may be different for each bacteria-plasmid system; therefore it needs to be determined in advance.

15. Although Eppendorf tubes can be used instead of cryo-tubes, snap-top tubes are usually not recommended as they can open unexpectedly at –80 °C. Label both the lid and the tube, because samples stored for long periods at –80 °C can lose labels stuck to the tube.

16. Before freezing the tubes, make sure there is uniform solution with no layers present. Bacteria viability decreases with repeated freezing-thawing cycles. Since this experiment requires that the inoculum contains a constant amount of viable bacteria, two glycerol stocks are advised in case one tube needs to be discarded.

17. Quantification of the percentage of bacteria containing pAmp in agar plates with and without Amp (Subheading 3.2) can be done either by starting from fresh daily cultures or from –80 °C thawed cultures.

18. Each culture may take 4–6 h to reach $OD_{600} = 0.5$. For this reason, this experiment is thought to be performed on consecutive convenient days.

19. To prepare 1/10 (10^{-1}) dilution in Eppendorf tubes, transfer 100 μl of G0 culture to 900 μl PBS (1×) and mix well with a vortex. For 10^{-2} dilution, transfer 100 μl of a 10^{-1} dilution to 900 μl PBS (1×), mix well, and proceed in the same way until a 10^{-6} dilution is achieved. The same serial dilutions can be prepared using a sterile 96-well plate (in this case, final volume will be 100 μl).

20. The number of CFU/ml in the original sample can be calculated with the following equation: CFU/ml original sample = CFU/plate × (1/ml aliquot plated) × dilution factor. For example, 95 colonies on a plate × 1/0.1 ml (aliquot) × 10^6 (dilution factor) = $9.5 × 10^8$ CFU/ml.

21. The suitable dilution for an *E. coli* culture at $OD_{600} = 0.5$ may be approximately 10^{-5}–10^{-6} in order to obtain 50–200 CFU/LB-agar plate. However, this dilution will be lower for unstable plasmids grown in Amp-LB-agar plates and needs to be estimated from the previous generation results.

Acknowledgments

I would like to thank Dr. Gloria del Solar and Dr. Manuel Espinosa (Center for Biological Research, Consejo Superior de Investigaciones Cientificas, Madrid, Spain) for having taught me this method in the early 90s. Thanks also to Dr. Jose A. Chabalgoity (Department of Biochemistry, School of Medicine, Universidad de la República, Montevideo, Uruguay) for his encouragement to write this chapter and to our undergraduate student, Rodrigo Gonzalez, for having tested this plasmid stability method in several Gram (–) host strains (Grant support: Comision Honoraria de Lucha Contra el Cáncer (CHLCC-Kramer 2009)).

References

1. Sambrook J, Russell DW (2001) Molecular cloning: a laboratory manual, 3rd edn. Cold Spring Harbor Laboratory press, New York. ISBN 0879695773
2. Kramer MG, Khan SA, Espinosa M (1997) Plasmid rolling circle replication: identification of the RNA polymerase-directed primer RNA and requirement for DNA polymerase I for lagging strand synthesis. EMBO J 16:5784–5795
3. Jensen RB, Dam M, Gerdes K (1994) Partitioning of plasmid R1. The parA operon is autoregulated by ParR and its transcription is highly stimulated by a downstream activating element. J Mol Biol 236:1299–1309
4. Sobecky PA, Easter CL, Bear PD, Helinski DR (1996) Characterization of the stable maintenance properties of the par region of broad-host-range plasmid RK2. J Bacteriol 178:2086–2093
5. Diago-Navarro E, Hernandez-Arriaga AM, López-Villarejo J, Muñoz-Gómez AJ, Kamphuis MB, Boelens R, Lemonnier M, Díaz-Orejas R (2010) parD toxin-antitoxin system of plasmid R1--basic contributions, biotechnological applications and relationships with closely-related toxin-antitoxin systems. FEBS J 277:3097–3117
6. Summers D (1998) Timing, self-control and a sense of direction are the secrets of multicopy plasmid stability. Mol Microbiol 29:1137–1145
7. del Solar G, Kramer G, Ballester S, Espinosa M (1993) Replication of the promiscuous plasmid pLS1: a region encompassing the minus origin of replication is associated with stable plasmid inheritance. Mol Gen Genet 241:97–105
8. Kramer MG, Espinosa M, Misra TK, Khan SA (1999) Characterization of a single-strand origin, ssoU, required for broad host range replication of rolling-circle plasmids. Mol Microbiol 33:466–475
9. Kramer MG, Espinosa M, Misra TK, Khan SA (1998) Lagging strand replication of rolling-circle plasmids: specific recognition of the ssoA-type origins in different gram-positive bacteria. Proc Natl Acad Sci U S A 95:10505–10510
10. Field CM, Summers DK (2011) Multicopy plasmid stability: revisiting the dimer catastrophe. J Theor Biol 291:119–127
11. Dunstan SJ, Simmons CP, Strugnell RA (2003) In vitro and in vivo stability of recombinant plasmids in a vaccine strain of Salmonella enterica var. Typhimurium. FEMS Immunol Med Microbiol 37:111–119
12. Bauer H, Darji A, Chakraborty T, Weiss S (2005) Salmonella-mediated oral DNA vaccination using stabilized eukaryotic expression plasmids. Gene Ther 12:364–372
13. Gahan ME, Webster DE, Wesselingh SL, Strugnell RA (2007) Impact of plasmid stability on oral DNA delivery by Salmonella enterica serovar Typhimurium. Vaccine 25:1476–1483
14. Moreno M, Kramer MG, Yim L, Chabalgoity JA (2010) Salmonella as live Trojan horse for vaccine development and cancer gene therapy. Curr Gene Ther 10:56–76
15. Kramer MG (2003) Orígenes de replicación de la cadena retrasada del plásmido pMV158 (Lagging-strand replication origins of plasmid pMV158). Universidad Complutense de Madrid (ed). ISBN: 9788466915298
16. Gonzalez R, Chabalgoity JA, and Kramer MG, unpublished results
17. Bertani G (1951) Studies on lysogenesis. I. The mode of phage liberation by lysogenic Escherichia coli. J Bacteriol 62:293–300
18. Luria SE, Burrous JW (1957) Hybridization between Escherichia coli and Shigella. J Bacteriol 74:461–476

Chapter 12

Visualization of Anticancer *Salmonella typhimurium* Engineered for Remote Control of Therapeutic Proteins

Vu H. Nguyen and Jung-Joon Min

Abstract

Tumor-targeting bacteria are studied for their ability to carry therapeutic molecules to tumors or, when designed as imaging probes, to visualize the infection pathway. The present protocol describes a method to achieve remote control of therapeutic gene expression in bacteria which are also engineered to visualize the therapeutic process. This strategy may increase the safety of bacteria used to deliver therapeutic genes to tumors in vivo.

Key words Bacteria, Cancer, Cytolysin A, pBAD, Imaging

1 Introduction

Attenuated *Salmonella typhimurium* is an effective tumor-targeting bacterial strain that accumulates naturally and replicates in a wide variety of solid tumors [1]. *S. typhimurium* bioengineered to generate bioluminescence [2, 3] or fluorescence [4] has been used to monitor bacterial migration to tumors in small-animal models. The signal may help predict the efficacy of bacteriolytic therapy by enabling the visualization of bacterial accumulation and replication in specific organs.

Here, attenuated *S. typhimurium*, which was defective in ppGpp synthesis (ΔppGpp strain), was engineered to express the cytotoxic protein, cytolysin A (ClyA), with the aim of killing cancer cells. The luciferase gene, *lux*, was integrated into the bacterial chromosome to allow noninvasive monitoring in vivo by detecting bioluminescence. Once the luminescence imaging signal showed that the bacteria had accumulated in the tumor and were cleared from normal organs, expression of the therapeutic gene was induced. This imageable therapeutic (theranostic) strategy can prevent toxicity to non-tumor reticuloendothelial organs, mainly the liver and spleen, in which the bacteria initially localized after tail vein injection [3, 5].

Robert M. Hoffman (ed.), *Bacterial Therapy of Cancer: Methods and Protocols*, Methods in Molecular Biology, vol. 1409,
DOI 10.1007/978-1-4939-3515-4_12, © Springer Science+Business Media New York 2016

2 Materials

2.1 Bacteria and Animals

1. Wild-type (WT) *S. typhimurium*.
2. *S. typhimurium* Xen26 (Xenogen, Caliper Life Sciences).
3. *S. typhimurium* harboring mutated *relA* and *spoT* genes (ΔppGpp *S. typhimurium*) [6].
4. WT *S. typhi*.
5. WT Phage 22.
6. Five- to six-week-old male BALB/c mice (Orient, Korea). All animal studies were conducted in accordance with standard animal-welfare regulations and were approved by the Chonnam National University Animal Care and Use Committee. Animals were maintained in ventilated chambers and fed an autoclaved laboratory rodent diet (PMI Nutrition, Brentwood, MO).

2.2 Reagents

1. SOC medium LB medium (Fisher Scientific, Tustin, CA).
2. pBAD-RLuc8 (a gift from Dr. Sam Gambhir, Stanford University, Stanford, CA).
3. Isoflurane (Abbott, Abbott Park, IL).
4. L-Arabinose (Sigma, St. Louis, MO).
5. Kanamycin (Amresco, Solon, OH).
6. Ampicillin (Sigma, St. Louis, MO).

2.3 Equipment

1. Syringes (Becton Dickinson, Franklin Lakes, NJ).
2. 0.22 μm syringe filter (Pall, MI).
3. 37 °C shaking incubator (SangWoo, Korea).
4. 37 °C incubator (Sanyo, Japan).
5. 0.2 cm gap electroporation cuvette (Bio-Rad, CA).
6. Gene Pulser apparatus (Bio-Rad Laboratories, Hercules, CA).
7. IVIS® Imaging System 100 (Caliper Life Sciences, Hopkinton, MA).
8. Living Image® 2.50.1 software (Caliper Life Sciences, Hopkinton, MA).

3 Methods

Carry out all the procedures at room temperature unless otherwise specified.

3.1 Establishing Luciferase-Expressing ΔppGpp S. typhimurium by Phage 22 Transduction

1. Inoculate 20 μl WT Phage 22 (P22) with 100 μl of an overnight culture of donor bacteria (*S. typhimurium* Xen26, Xenogen/Caliper Life Sciences) in a 1.5 ml centrifuge tube. Incubate the cells with agitation at 200 rpm (37 °C) overnight.

2. Add 100 µl chloroform into the tube, vortex for 1 min, centrifuge at $12,000 \times g$ for 10 min, transfer the supernatant to a new centrifuge tube, and then repeat once.

3. Transfer the supernatant containing P22 into a glass tube, add several drops of chloroform, cap tightly, and store at 4 °C (*see* **Note 1**).

4. Mix 100 µl of the recipient-cell suspension (ΔppGpp *S. typhimurium*) from the overnight culture with 20 µl of P22 suspension.

5. Incubate these suspensions at 37 °C for 1 h.

6. Spread all the transduced bacteria or 100 µl non-transduced bacteria or 20 µl P22 suspension (negative controls) onto LB plates containing 50 mg/ml kanamycin. Incubate in a 37 °C incubator with the lid down.

7. Select transductants (*S.typhimurium* Lux) by observing luciferase expression (light emitting) with a cooled CCD camera.

8. Select a single light-emitting colony and transfer it to liquid LB medium containing kanamycin.

9. Incubate at 37 °C overnight and store at –80 °C using a 20 % final concentration of glycerol.

3.2 Construction of the Inducible ClyA Expression Plasmid

1. Amplify the *clyA* gene with 5′-AGT CCA TGG TTA TGA CCG GAA TAT TTG C-3′ (forward primer) and 5′-GAT GTT TAA ACT CAG ACG TCA GGA ACC TC-3′ (reverse primer) using *S. typhi* genomic DNA as a template [7].

2. Digest the amplified DNA with *NcoI* and *PmeI* and replace RLuc8 with ClyA by ligation. The expression plasmid pBAD-RLuc8 has been described previously [8].

3. Confirm ClyA expression under control of the pBAD promoter by hemolytic activity assay using sheep blood agar plates (*see* **Note 2**) (Fig. 1).

3.3 Generation of ΔppGpp S. typhimurium Expressing Luciferase (S.t.Lux) with a Remote-Controlled Expression System

1. Prepare a fresh 1 % bacterial culture (assessed by OD_{600}) from an overnight bacterial culture in LB medium. Incubate the cells with agitation at 200 rpm (37 °C).

2. When the bacteria reach mid-log phase, harvest the cells by cooled centrifugation at $2500 \times g$ for 5 min (4 °C).

3. Wash the cells three times with ice-cold glycerol (10 % vol/vol in purified water) and resuspend them in ice-cold glycerol (10 % vol/vol) at a volume approximately 1:100 that of the original culture volume.

4. Transfer 80 µl of the bacterial solution (approximately 10^8 cells) in ice-cold glycerol to a 0.2 cm gap electroporation cuvette.

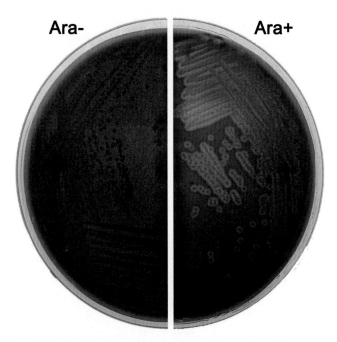

Ara-   **Ara+**

Fig. 1 *S.typhimurium* lux pBC was streaked onto a sheep blood agar plate without L-arabinose (*left*) or with 0.2 % L-arabinose (*right*) for overnight incubation at 37 °C

5. Add 10 ng pBAD-ClyA (pBC) to the bacterial suspension and mix gently.

6. Electroporate the cells at 1.8 kV for 1 s using the Gene Pulser apparatus according to the manufacturer's instructions.

7. Add 1 ml of SOC medium to the cuvette immediately after the electric pulse.

8. Transfer the bacterial suspension into a fresh 15 ml polypropylene tube and incubate the cells at 37 °C with agitation at 200 rpm for 45 min.

9. Inoculate LB agar plates containing ampicillin and kanamycin with 200 μl of the bacterial suspension using the spreading technique.

10. Incubate the plates overnight at 37 °C.

11. Select a single colony (*S.typhimurium* Lux + pBC) and transfer it to liquid LB medium containing ampicillin and kanamycin.

12. Incubate at 37 °C overnight and store at –80 °C using a 20 % final concentration of glycerol.

3.4 Growth of Bacteria for Infection in Living Mice

1. Select a single bacterial colony from an LB agar plate containing ampicillin and kanamycin and inoculate a 5 ml liquid LB culture containing the same antibiotics.

2. Incubate the inoculated tube in a shaking incubator overnight at 37 °C.

3. Prepare a fresh 1 % culture of the overnight bacterial suspension in LB medium containing the same antibiotics and incubate the cells in a shaking incubator (37 °C, 200 rpm) for 3–4 h until the bacteria reach early-stationary phase ($OD_{600} \sim 3.0$–3.5).

4. Harvest fresh bacterial cultures (in early stationary phase), wash the cells with sterile phosphate-buffered saline (PBS), and estimate bacterial number with a spectrophotometer (OD_{600}). Suspend cells in PBS at the desired concentration.

5. Anesthetize mice in a chamber ventilated with isoflurane and oxygen (*see* **Note 3**).

6. Administer bacteria (4.5×10^7 CFU suspended in 100 µl PBS) by lateral tail vein injection using a 1 ml latex-free syringe fitted with a 31-gauge needle (Becton Dickinson) (*see* **Note 4**).

3.5 Whole-Body Imaging with the IVIS

1. Anesthetize mice in a chamber ventilated with isoflurane and oxygen.

2. Place the mice into the IVIS chamber with their noses ventilated by anesthetic gas conducted through tubes protruding into the chamber.

3. Close the chamber tightly and begin acquiring images as described in the whole-body imaging equipment section (*see* **Note 5**) (Fig. 2).

4. Capture the luminescence emitted from the mice with the camera and evaluate it using Living Image® software (*see* **Note 6**).

3.6 Induction of the Gene Under the Control of the pBAD Promoter

1. Dilute L-arabinose (Sigma) in PBS to obtain 40 % (w/vol) final concentration and then sterilize using a 0.22 µm syringe filter.

2. To induce gene expression, 60 mg or 120 mg L-arabinose, diluted in filtered-sterile PBS, can be administered intravenously or intraperitoneally, respectively (*see* **Note 7**) (Fig. 3).

4 Notes

1. The chloroform in the P22 suspension helps to prevent bacterial contamination.

2. In the new vector, pBAD-ClyA, the *clyA* gene is controlled by an L-arabinose-inducible promoter. Therefore, sheep blood

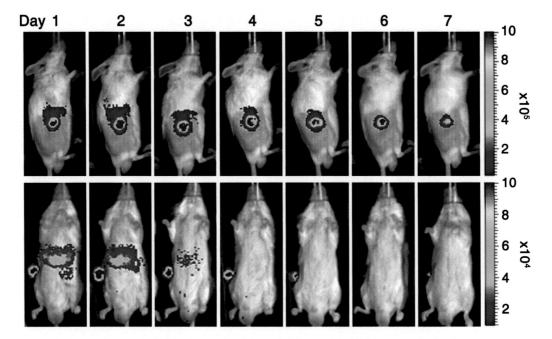

Fig. 2 Noninvasive in vivo imaging of bacterial bioluminescence in representative tumor-bearing mice. Mice with the CT-26 murine colon cancer tumor were treated with *S. typhimurium* Lux + pBC. Each bacterium carries the lux operon in its chromosome. The lux operon encodes all proteins required for bioluminescence, including bacterial luciferase, substrate, and substrate-regenerating enzymes. The bacteria engineered to express the *lux* operon do not require an exogenous substrate to produce bioluminescence. In order to image bacterial bioluminescence, anesthetized animals were placed in the light-tight chamber of the IVIS-100, equipped with a cooled CCD camera. Photons emitted from lux-expressing bacteria were collected and integrated over 1 min periods. Pseudo-color images indicating photon counts were overlaid on photographs of the mice using Living Image software v. 2.25. Photon intensity was recorded as the maximum intensity (photons·s^{-1} cm^{-2} sr^{-1})

agar plates with or without L-arabinose can be used to confirm the induction of ClyA expression.

3. After injecting the bacteria, anesthetized mice can be imaged immediately using the IVIS to confirm the success of injection. Mice are then imaged daily for the duration of the experiment to visualize the location of bacteria.

4. If it is hard to see the vein, dip the tail in warm water (37–40 °C) 1 min before injection.

5. The exposure time, f-stop setting, and binning values should be kept constant for every image to avoid inconsistent analyses.

6. The light emitted from bacteria can be absorbed by the hair of the mice, so removal of the hair before imaging is suggested.

7. Induction is started when most of the bacteria have been cleared in the normal organs, such as the liver and spleen. In this study, gene expression was induced from day 4 after injection of bacteria.

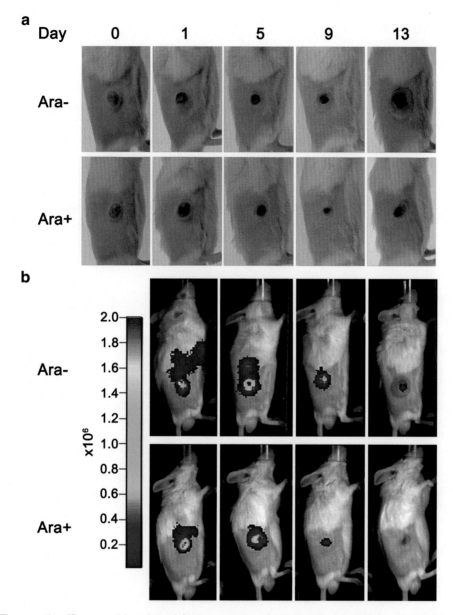

Fig. 3 Therapeutic efficacy and imaging of ClyA-expressing *S. typhimurium* in CT26 murine colon cancer-bearing mice. BALB/c mice ($n = 5$ in each group) were injected subcutaneously with CT-26 cells. After tumors reached 130 mm^3 in volume, tumor-bearing mice were treated with transformed *S. typhimurium* bearing pBAD-ClyA plasmid (*S. typhimurium* Lux +pBC). ClyA gene expression was induced (Ara+) with 60 mg L-arabinose by intravenous injection every day, beginning 4 days post injection of bacteria. The non-induced group (Ara−) was used as a control. (**a**) Photographs of subcutaneous tumors in representative mice. (**b**) Noninvasive in vivo imaging of bacterial bioluminescence in the representative mice presented in (**a**)

Acknowledgments

This research was supported by the Bio R&D program of the Korea Science and Engineering Foundation (KOSEF) funded by the Ministry of Education, Science and Technology (MEST, 2008-04131), the National Research Foundation of Korea (NRF) funded by the Ministry of Education, Science and Technology (No. 2009-0091729), the National R&D Program for Cancer Control, Ministry of Health & Welfare, Republic of Korea (0620330-1), and in part by the BioImaging Research Center at GIST. Y.H. was supported by grant no. RTI05-01-01 from the Regional Technology Innovation Program of the Ministry of Commerce, Industry and Energy (MOCIE), and H.E.C. was supported by a KOSEF grant funded by MEST (No. 2007-04213).

References

1. Pawelek JM, Low KB, Bermudes D (2003) Bacteria as tumour-targeting vectors. Lancet Oncol 4:548–556

2. Min JJ, Nguyen VH, Kim HJ et al (2008) Quantitative bioluminescence imaging of tumor-targeting bacteria in living animals. Nat Protoc 3:629–636

3. Yu YA, Shabahang S, Timiryasova TM et al (2004) Visualization of tumors and metastases in live animals with bacteria and vaccinia virus encoding light-emitting proteins. Nat Biotechnol 22:313–320

4. Hoffman RM, Zhao M (2006) Whole-body imaging of bacterial infection and antibiotic response. Nat Protoc 1:2988–2994

5. Min JJ, Kim HJ, Park JH et al (2008) Noninvasive real-time imaging of tumors and metastases using tumor-targeting light-emitting Escherichia coli. Mol Imaging Biol 10:54–61

6. Nguyen VH, Kim HS, Ha JM et al (2010) Genetically engineered Salmonella typhimurium as an imageable therapeutic probe for cancer. Cancer Res 70:18–23

7. Piao HH, Seong J, Song MK et al (2009) The bacterial surface expression of SARS viral epitope using Salmonella typhi Cytolysin A. J Bacteriol Virol 39:103–112

8. Loening AM, Fenn TD, Wu AM et al (2006) Consensus guided mutagenesis of Renilla luciferase yields enhanced stability and light output. Protein Eng Des Sel 19:391–400

Chapter 13

Methods for Tumor Targeting with *Salmonella typhimurium* A1-R

Robert M. Hoffman and Ming Zhao

Abstract

Salmonella typhimurium A1-R (*S. typhimurium* A1-R) has shown great preclinical promise as a broad-based anti-cancer therapeutic (please *see* Chapter 1). The present chapter describes materials and methods for the preclinical study of *S. typhimurium* A1-R in clinically-relevant mouse models. Establishment of orthotopic metastatic mouse models of the major cancer types is described, as well as other useful models, for efficacy studies of *S. typhimurium* A1-R or other tumor-targeting bacteria, as well. Imaging methods are described to visualize GFP-labeled *S. typhimurium* A1-R, as well as GFP- and/or RFP-labeled cancer cells in vitro and in vivo, which *S. typhimurium* A1-R targets. The mouse models include metastasis to major organs that are life-threatening to cancer patients including the liver, lung, bone, and brain and how to target these metastases with *S. typhimurium* A1-R. Various routes of administration of *S. typhimurium* A1-R are described with the advantages and disadvantages of each. Basic experiments to determine toxic effects of *S. typhimurium* A1-R are also described. Also described are methodologies for combining *S. typhimurium* A1-R and chemotherapy. The testing of *S. typhimurium* A1-R on patient tumors in patient-derived orthotopic xenograft (PDOX) mouse models is also described. The major methodologies described in this chapter should be translatable for clinical studies.

Key words *Salmonella typhimurium* A1-R, Tumor targeting, Leu-Arg, Amino acid, Auxotroph, Green fluorescent protein (GFP), Surgical orthotopic implantation (SOI), Nude mice, Mouse models, Cancer, Metastasis, Orthotopic

1 Introduction

Salmonella typhimurium A1-R (*S. typhimurium* A1-R), developed in our laboratory, is a facultative anaerobe that can live and replicate in viable as well as necrotic areas of tumors. *S. typhimurium* A1-R is auxotrophic for Leu-Arg which prevents it from mounting a continuous infection in normal tissues. *S. typhimurium* A1-R has no other known attenuating mutations and has been further selected for high tumor virulence. *S. typhimurium* A1-R was able to inhibit primary and metastatic tumors in monotherapy in nude mouse models of major types of human cancer [1].

Robert M. Hoffman (ed.), *Bacterial Therapy of Cancer: Methods and Protocols*, Methods in Molecular Biology, vol. 1409, DOI 10.1007/978-1-4939-3515-4_13, © Springer Science+Business Media New York 2016

In a phase I clinical trial on patients with metastatic melanoma and renal carcinoma, the *S. typhimurium* strain tested (VNP20009), attenuated by msbB and purI mutations, was safely administered to patients. However, VNP20009 did not sufficiently colonize the patients' tumors, perhaps because this strain was over-attenuated [2] or was not sufficiently selected for tumor virulence [3]. *S. typhimurium* A1-R has higher tumor colonization efficiency and anti-tumor efficacy than VNP20009, which has more attenuating mutations than *S. typhimurium* A1-R [4].

S. typhimurium A1-R was able to strongly inhibit primary and metastatic tumors as monotherapy in nude mouse models of ovarian [5, 6], prostate [7, 8], breast [3, 9, 10], lung [4, 11, 12], and pancreatic [13, 14] cancers, as well as sarcoma [15–17] and glioma [18, 19], all of which are highly aggressive tumor models. *S. typhimurium* A1-R also targeted pancreatic cancer stem-like cells [20] and pancreatic cancer patient-derived orthotopic xenograft (PDOX) models [21, 22]. We have recently demonstrated that *S. typhimurium* A1-R prevents breast cancer bone and brain metastasis in nude mouse models [9, 10].

This chapter presents methods for evaluating the efficacy of *S.typhimurium* A1-R in mouse models of cancer.

2 Materials

2.1 Reagents

1. LB medium (Life Technologies).
2. SOC medium (Life Technologies).
3. Fetal bovine serum (Gemini Biol. Products).
4. Lipofectamine PLUS (Invitrogen).
5. G418 neomycin (Invitrogen).
6. Kanamycin (Life Technologies).
7. pGFP (Clontech).
8. *EGFP* gene (Clontech).
9. RFP cDNA (pDsRed2; Clontech).
10. Plasmid pLNCX2 (Clontech).
11. Supernatants of PT67-GFP cells, PT67-RFP cells, and PT67 H2B-GFP cells (Clontech).
12. PT67 packaging cells (Clontech).
13. Restriction enzymes HindIII and NotI (Life Technologies).
14. Anesthetic reagents (ketamine, xylazine, acepromazine maleate) (Henry Schein).
15. Matrigel (BD Bioscience).
16. Nair (Church & Dwight).

17. *E. coli*; JM 109 (Stratagene).

18. *S. typhimurium* 14028 (American Type Culture Collection).

19. Growth medium (normal and selective) appropriate for cell culture, such as DMEM (Invitrogen; Irvine Scientific).

20. Polybrene (Sigma Aldrich).

21. Trypsin-EDTA (Fisher Scientific).

22. Non-transgenic and transgenic nude (nu/nu) mice expressing GFP or RFP (AntiCancer Inc.).

23. Doxorubicin (Pharmaceutical Buyers International).

24. NaCl, 0.9 % (Sigma Aldrich).

25. Optimum cutting temperature compound (OCT) (VWR).

26. Antibody to rat immunoglobulin (anti-rat immunoglobulin) and anti-mouse immunoglobulin horseradish peroxidase detection kits (BD PharMingen).

27. Monoclonal anti-CD31 (CBL1337; Chemicon).

28. Monoclonal anti-nestin (rat 401; BD PharMingen).

29. Substrate-chromogen 3,3′-diaminobenzidine (Sigma Aldrich).

30. C57BL/6 and Balb/c mice (AntiCancer Inc.).

31. Fluorescent protein-expressing cancer cell lines (AntiCancer, Inc.).

32. TNF-α enzyme-linked immunosorbent assay (ELISA) kit (Invitrogen).

2.2   Equipment

1. 1-ml 27G2 latex-free syringe (Becton Dickinson).

2. 25-μl Hamilton syringe (Sigma Aldrich).

3. Hemocytometer (Sigma Aldrich).

4. 28-G latex-free insulin syringe (0.5 ml 28 G) (TYCO Health Group LP).

5. Gene Pulser apparatus (Bio-Rad Laboratories).

6. Culture dishes, 60 mm; flask, 25 mm; plates, 96-well (Fisher Scientific).

7. Cloning cylinders (Sigma Aldrich).

8. 27G2 latex-free syringe, 1 ml (Becton Dickinson).

9. 8-0 surgical sutures (Sutures Express).

10. Humidified incubator with an atmosphere of 5 % CO_2 (Thermo Scientific).

11. Blue LED flashlight (LDP LLC).

12. D470/40 excitation filter (Chroma Technology).

13. GG475 emission filter (Chroma Technology).

14. Fluorescence light box with fiber-optic lighting at 470 nm (Lightools Fluorescent Imaging System; Lightools Research).

15. CM1850 cryostat (Leica).

16. LZ12 fluorescence stereo microscope (Leica).

17. MZ6 stereo microscope (Leica).

18. Multiphoton tomography MPT*flex*™ (JenLab GmbH and MultiPhoton Laser Technologies Inc.).

19. BH 2-RFCA fluorescence microscope equipped with a mercury 100-W lamp power supply (Olympus Corp.).

20. OV100 Small Animal Imaging System, containing an MT-20 light source and DP70 CCD camera (Olympus).

21. IV100 Laser Scanning Imaging System (Olympus).

22. FluoView FV1000 Confocal Microscope (Olympus).

23. Illumatool instrument (Lightools Research).

24. iBox Scientia Imaging System (UVP, LLC).

25. Maestro fluorescence imaging system (CRi, Perkin-Elmer Inc.)

26. Hamamatsu C5810 three-chip cooled color CCD camera (Hamamatsu Photonics Systems).

27. Image-Pro Plus 4.0 software (Media Cybernetics).

28. Paint Shop Pro 8 (Corel).

29. CellR (Olympus).

30. Coolpix camera (Nikon).

---

3   Methods

3.1   GFP Labeling of S. typhimurium (See Note 1)

1. Mix bacteria cells (2.0×10^8) with 10 % glycerol and 2 μl pGFP (Clontech).

2. To transform *S. typhimurium* with the GFP gene, perform electroporation with a Gene Pulser apparatus (Bio-Rad) at 1.8 kV with the pulse controller at 1000-W parallel resistance.

3.2   Induction of Mutations with Nitrosoguanidine (NTG) and Selection for Auxotrophs (See Notes 2–5)

1. Add freshly prepared NTG (1 mg/ml in sterile water) to a washed bacterial culture to a final concentration of 100 μg/ml in Tris-maleic acid buffer at pH 6.0.

2. Incubate the bacteria with NTG for 30 min.

3. Grow the NTG-treated bacteria in nutrient broth to express any mutations that were induced. Replica plate bacterial colonies in supplemented minimal agar plates containing specific amino acids to identify the requirements of the auxotrophs.

4. Identify the auxotrophic amino acids such as for *S. typhimurium* A1, which requires Leu and Arg.

3.3 Selection of High Tumor-Targeting Strain, S. typhimurium A1-R (See Notes 6 and 7)

Select high tumor-targeting substrain of *S. typhimurium* A1 expressing GFP as follows:

1. Inject *S. typhimurium* A1 into the tail vein of a HT-29 human colon tumor-bearing nude mouse.

2. Remove the tumor tissue from the infected mouse after 3 days.

3. Homogenize the tumor tissue and dilute with PBS. Culture the supernatant resulting from centrifugation of the homogenized tumor tissue in LB agar plates at 37 °C overnight.

4. Pick the bacteria colony with the brightest green fluorescence and culture in 5 ml LB medium. This strain was termed *S. typhimurium* A1-R [3].

3.4 Adherence and Invasion Assay for Comparison Between S. typhimurium A1 and A1-R

1. Grow RFP-labeled HT-29 human colon cancer cells in 24-well tissue culture plates to a density of ~10^4 cells per well.

2. Grow *S. typhimurium* A1-R to late-log phase in LB broth [7].

3. Dilute the bacteria in cell culture medium and add to the cancer cells, then place in an incubator at 37 °C. After 60 min, rinse the cells five times with 1–2-ml PBS.

4. Incubate with 0.2 ml 0.1 % Triton X-100 for 10 min to release adherent bacteria. Add LB broth (0.8 ml) and mix each sample vigorously.

5. Quantify adherent bacteria by plating in order to count colony-forming units (CFU) on LB agar medium.

6. To measure cancer cell invasion of bacteria, rinse the bacterially-infected cancer cells five times with 1–2 ml PBS and culture in medium containing gentamicin sulfate (20 μg/ml) to kill external, but not internal, bacteria.

7. Wash the cells once with PBS after incubation with gentamicin for 12 h and image the viable intracellular bacteria with fluorescence microscopy [3].

3.5 Invasiveness of Dual-Color Cancer Cells by S. typhimurium A1-R (See Note 8)

1. Grow dual-color PC-3 human prostate cancer cells labeled with RFP in the cytoplasm and in the nucleus with GFP fused to histone H2B in 24-well tissue culture plates.

2. Grow *S. typhimurium* A1-R in LB medium and harvest at late-log phase, then dilute in cell culture medium and add to the cancer cells.

3. Rinse the cells and culture in medium containing gentamicin sulfate to kill external, but not internal, bacteria after 1 h of incubation at 37 °C.

4. Observe the interaction between *S. typhimurium* A1-R and cancer cells under fluorescence microscopy. Visualize the

bacteria in the cancer cells undergoing rapid apoptosis by fragmentation of the GFP-expressing nuclei [3].

3.6 Confocal Imaging of Cancer Cells Infected with S. typhimurium A1-R

1. For high-resolution imaging of cancer cells infected with *S. typhimurium* in vitro and in vivo, use a confocal microscope (FluoView FV1000, Olympus) [23].

2. Obtain fluorescence images using the 20×/0.50 UPLAN FLN and 40×/1.3 oil Olympus UPLAN FLN objectives [24].

3.7 Surgical Orthotopic Implantation (SOI) of Breast Tumors

1. Anesthetize 4–6-week-old nude mice with a ketamine mixture (10 μl ketamine HCL, 7.6 μl xylazine, 2.4 μl acepromazine maleate and 10 μl H_2O) via s.c. injection. Implant tumor fragments (1 mm^3), harvested from the MARY-X human breast tumor or other breast tumors [25] previously grown s.c. in nude mice, by surgical orthotopic implantation (SOI) in the mammary fat pad in 4–6-week-old female nude mice. Use 8-0 surgical sutures to attach the tumor pieces to the fat pad.

2. Close the incision in the skin with a 6-0 surgical suture in one layer. Keep the mice under isoflurane anesthesia during surgery [3].

3.8 Bacterial Targeting of Experimental Lung Metastasis (See Note 9)

1. Use 4–6-week-old nude mice.

2. Inject 143B-RFP human osteosarcoma cells (1×10^6 in 100 μl PBS) into the tail vein of nude mice to obtain experimental lung metastasis.

3. On day 7, 14, and 21, inject 5×10^7 *S. typhimurium* A1-R CFU per mouse into the tail vein.

4. On day 28, sacrifice all animals and image the excised lungs with the Olympus OV100 Small Animal Imaging System (0.14× lens, excitation 535–555 nm, emission 570–623 nm) or similar fluorescence imaging system and count the number of metastases [16].

3.9 Orthotopic Osteosarcoma Model in Nude Mice

1. Anesthetize 4–6-week-old nude mice with the ketamine mixture (described above) via s.c. injection. Sterilize the leg with alcohol and make a 2 mm midline skin incision just below the knee joint to expose the tibial tuberosity [16].

2. Inject 5×10^5 RFP-expressing 143B-RFP cells in 5 μl Matrigel per mouse into the intramedullary cavity of the tibia with a 0.5 ml 28-G latex-free insulin syringe.

3. Close the skin with a 6-0 suture.

4. One week after injection, make a 1-cm skin incision over the tibia to confirm that the RFP tumor is growing inside of the bone using the OV100 or similar imaging system and then close the skin again as described above [16].

3.10 S. typhimurium A1-R Therapy of Experimental Pancreatic Cancer Lymph-Node Metastasis (See Notes 10 and 11)

1. To obtain metastasis in the axillary lymph node, inject XPA-1-RFP human pancreatic cancer cells into the inguinal lymph node (afferent lymph node to the axillary) in 4–6-week-old nude mice.

2. Anesthetize nude mice with the ketamine mixture (described above) via s.c. injection.

3. Make a 1 cm incision in the abdominal skin to expose the inguinal lymph node. Expose the inguinal lymph node without injuring the lymphatic. Fix the skin on a flat stand with pins. Inject a total of 10 μl medium containing 5×10^5 cancer cells into the center of the inguinal lymph node.

4. Seven days later (day 0), anesthetize the mice and observe the axillary lymph node for metastasis. Make a 2 cm incision at the center of the chest wall. Release the greater pectoral muscle from the sternum to expose the axillary lymph node. Separate the connective tissue on the axillary lymph node. Image the lymph node for metastasis.

5. Inject *S. typhimurium* A1-R (10^8 CFU [use a lower dose if toxicity is observed]) in the inguinal lymph node.

6. After injection, observe the axillary lymph node repeatedly at different time points with the OV100 or similar imaging system. Measure the size of metastasis (fluorescent area [mm²]) at each imaging time point [15].

3.11 S. typhimurium A1-R Therapy of Spontaneous Lymph-Node Metastasis

1. To obtain spontaneous lymph node metastasis, inject 5×10^6 HT-1080-GFP-RFP human fibrosarcoma cells in 20 μl Matrigel into the footpad in 4–6-week-old nude mice.

2. Determine the presence of popliteal lymph node metastasis by fluorescence imaging every week after cancer-cell injection. Anesthetize the mice with the ketamine mixture (described above) and lay out in a prone position.

3. Observe the entire limb with the OV100 imaging system non-invasively. Start bacteria therapy, targeting the metastasis (day 0), once metastasis is confirmed in the popliteal region.

4. Inject *S. typhimurium* A1-R (10^8 CFU [use a lower dose if toxicity is observed]) subcutaneously in the footpad. Measure the size of metastasis and primary tumor and body weight every week. Treat 6 mice with *S. typhimurium* A1-R and use another 6 mice as controls. Use another two mice for imaging immediately and at day 7 after *S. typhimurium* A1-R injection. Terminate the experiment when the untreated control primary tumor invades the popliteal region or when the mouse died [15].

3.12 Intra-tumoral Bacterial Therapy for Pancreatic Cancer (See Note 12)

1. Surgically expose the tumor on day 7 after orthotopic implantation and image with the OV100 or similar imaging system. Measure the size of the tumor (fluorescent area [mm²]).

2. Treat three mice intra-tumorally (i.t.) with a low concentration of *S. typhimurium* A1-R (10^7 CFU/ml), treat 3 mice i.t. with a high concentration (10^8 CFU/ml), and use 3 as untreated controls.

3. Calculate tumor volume (mm³) with the formula $V = 1/2 \times$ (length × width²).

4. Expose the tumor again on day 14 and measure the size to determine the efficacy of treatment [13].

3.13 Selection of Highly Aggressive Subpopulations of XPA-1-RFP Human Pancreatic Cancer Cells

1. Serially-passage XPA-1-RFP human pancreatic cancer cells in the pancreas of 4–6-week-old nude mice.

2. Sacrifice the mice after they develop disseminated disease, including malignant ascites, and inject 50 μl of ascitic fluid into the pancreas of another nude mouse.

3. After five successive passages, transfer the ascitic fluid from the final passage into a cell-culture flask containing RPMI 1640 supplemented with 10 % FBS, 2 mM glutamine with 1 % penicillin-streptomycin. Place the flasks at 37 °C in a 5 % CO_2 incubator.

4. After the cancer cells are adherent, maintain the cells in culture as described above. This highly aggressive subpopulation of XPA-1-RFP human pancreatic cancer cells is henceforth referred to as XPA-1-RFP P5A.

5. Harvest mesenteric metastases from the same fifth-generation animal and fragment the tumor with surgical instruments and place in a cell culture dish with RPMI 1640 supplemented with 10 % fetal bovine serum, 2 mM glutamine with 1 % penicillin-streptomycin. Store the flasks at 37 °C in a 5 % incubator.

6. Once adherent cancer cells are detected via microscopy, passage the cells and maintain in culture as described above. This second population of highly aggressive XPA-1-RFP human pancreatic cancer cells is henceforth referred to as XPA-1-RFP P5B [14].

3.14 Intrasplenic Injection of Pancreatic Cancer Cells (See Note 13)

1. Anesthetize 4–6-week-old nude mice with the ketamine mixture (described above) injected subcutaneously.

2. Inject human XPA-1-RFP P5 A or B pancreatic cancer cells ($5.0 \times 10^6/50$ μl Matrigel) slowly as a cell suspension into the spleen of nude mice during open laparotomy. Secure hemostasis by gentle pressure using surgical gauze for 2 min.

3. Suture the skin and peritoneum in a single layer using 6-0 Prolene sutures [14].

3.15 Dose-Response of S. typhimurium A1-R Treatment of Metastatic Pancreatic Cancer

1. Treat nude mice with XPA-1 pancreatic cancer with either a low concentration of *S. typhimurium* A1-R (10^7 CFU/ml) or high concentration (10^8 CFU/ml) or do not treat (untreated control).

3.16 Orthotopic Transplantation of RFP-Expressing U87 Human Glioma for an Intramedullary Spinal Cord Tumor (IMSCT) Model

1. For an orthotopic intramedullary spinal cord tumor (IMSCT) model, harvest tumor fragments (0.5 mm) from subcutaneously growing U87-RFP human glioma tumors and implant by SOI into the spinal cord.

2. Make a midline incision approximately 2 cm long over the midthoracic spine. Perform sub-periosteal dissection of the para-vertebral muscles.

3. Remove the spinous process and bilateral lamina at the mid-thoracic level (T-7) using a blade to expose the dura mater.

4. Insert a 28-G needle into the dorsal center of the spinal cord, avoiding blood vessel injury, to create a 1-mm longitudinal incision.

5. Select the tumor pieces for implantation by RFP expression.

6. Implant U87-RFP tumor fragments into the incision of the spinal cord.

7. Close the muscles, fascia, and skin with a 6-0 surgical suture. After recovery, return the animals to their cages [18].

3.17 S. typhimurium A1-R Therapy of the Orthotopic IMSCT Model (See Note 14)

1. Five and ten days after transplantation of tumors, treat mice with *S. typhimurium* A1-R (2×10^7 CFU / 200 µl *i.v.* injection or 2×10^6 CFU / 10 µl intrathecal injection).

2. For intrathecal injection, anesthetize the mice and place on a sterile field. Identify the prominent L7 spinous process through palpation of the iliac crest and make a 0.5-cm longitudinal incision over the dorsal lower-lumber region.

3. Sweep the underlying fascia laterally and remove the spinous process at L7 and the ligamentum flavum to expose the intervertebral space.

4. Insert a 33-gauge 1/2-in. removable needle connected to a 10-µl syringe (Hamilton, Reno, NV) through the dorsal L6–L7 intervertebral space.

5. Treat eight mice with *S. typhimurium* A1-R via i.v. injection of 8 mice via intrathecal injection, and use 8 mice for an untreated control group [18].

3.18 Functional Evaluation of Hind Limbs to Determine Degree of Paralysis in the IMSCT Model Treated with *S. typhimurium*

1. Assess functional evaluation of hind limb strength using the Basso, Bresnahan, and Beattie (BBB) scale [26]. Place mice in an open-field testing area and observe for 5 min. Rate locomotion using the BBB locomotor scale. The BBB scale ranges from 21 to 0 (21 means consistent plantar stepping and coordinated gait, consistent toe clearance, predominant paw position parallel throughout stance, consistent trunk stability, and tail consistently up. Zero means no observable hind limb movement). Test all animals preoperatively to ensure a baseline locomotor rating of 21.

2. After tumor transplantation, test the animals three times a week. Assign two different observers randomly to score the animals' motor function. Results of the BBB score are expressed as the mean. Conclude the experiment by day 30 and sacrifice all animals at that time. Record dead animals in each group with a zero (0) functional score [18].

3.19 Treatment of RFP-Expressing Murine Lung Cancer Mouse Model Implanted at Various Sites (See Note 15)

1. Use ten nestin-driven GFP (ND-GFP) transgenic nude mice, 6–8-weeks-old.

2. Anesthetize mice with tribromoethanol (i.p. injection 0.2 ml/10 g body weight of a 1.2 % solution).

3. Inject RFP-expressing Lewis lung carcinoma (LLC) murine lung cancer cells (2×10^7 cells/ml) into the skin of the ear, back, and footpad of the ND-GFP nude mice with a 1 ml 27G1/2 latex-free syringe, 25 μl each site [12].

4. Treat mice with *S. typhimurium* A1-R via tail vein injection [12].

3.20 Efficacy of *S. typhimurium* A1-R on Experimental Lewis Lung Carcinoma Metastasis in the Lungs of C57 Mice

1. Use female C57 immuno-competent mice, age 6 weeks.

2. Inject RFP-expressing LLC cells (2×10^6 in 100 μl PBS) into the tail vein of C57 mice.

3. For treatment of LLC cells growing in the lung, administer either a single high dose (5×10^7 bacteria) or a medium dose, 2×10^7 CFU per mouse, by weekly injection or a low metronomic dose (1×10^7 CFU) per mouse twice a week i.v.

4. Administer *S. typhimurium* A1-R (1×10^8 CFU [use a lower dose if toxicity is observed]) in the thorax [24].

3.21 Craniotomy Open Window

1. Anesthetize the mice with the ketamine mixture (described above) via s.c. injection.

2. After fixing the mice in a prone position, make a 1.5 cm incision directly down the midline of the scalp. Retract the scalp and expose the skull. Using a skin biopsy punch, make a 4-mm diameter craniotomy over the right parietal bone.

3. Remove bone fragment carefully in order not to injure the meninges and brain tissue. Cover the craniotomy open window only with the scalp.

4. Inject U87-RFP cells (2×10^5) into the mouse brain via the craniotomy open window to a depth of 1 mm using a Hamilton syringe [19].

5. Close the incision with a 6-0 surgical suture.

6. Retract the scalp over the craniotomy window in order to image tumor growth in the brain.

7. Keep all mice in an oxygenated warmed chamber until they recover from anesthesia [19].

3.22   S. typhimurium A1-R Therapy in the Brain Tumor Model (See Note 16)

1. Two weeks after cancer-cell inoculation, treat mice with *S. typhimurium* A1-R (2×10^7 CFU / 200 μl PBS i.v. or 1×10^6 CFU/1 μl PBS through the craniotomy open window into the cranium) once a week for 3 weeks.

2. Administer the same volume of PBS to the un-treated control mice.

3. After administration of *S. typhimurium* A1-R, perform fluorescence imaging with the OV100 or similar imaging system and record changes in the diameter of the RFP-expressing brain tumors each week for 3 weeks.

4. Measure tumor diameter each week after *S. typhimurium* A1-R administration.

5. Calculate tumor volume with the formula (width$^2 \times$ length $\times$ 0.5). Use seven mice in each group [19].

3.23   Targeting MDA-MB-435-GFP-RFP Breast Cancer Cells with S. typhimurium A1-R In Vitro

1. Grow dual-color MDA-MB-435 cells, labeled with GFP in the nucleus and RFP in the cytoplasm, on 24-well tissue culture plates to a density of 10^4 cells per well.

2. Grow *S. typhimurium* A1-R in LB medium and harvest at late-log phase, then dilute in cell culture medium and add to the cancer cells [1×10^5 CFU per cell].

3. After 1 h incubation at 37 °C, rinse the cells and culture in medium containing gentamicin sulfate (20 μg/ml), to kill external, but not internal, *S. typhimurium* A1-R.

4. Observe the interaction between *S. typhimurium* A1-R and cancer cells, including apoptosis indicated by nuclear fragmentation, at different time points using the Olympus FluoView FV1000 confocal or other fluorescence microscope [27].

3.24   Mammary Fat Pad Orthotopic Injection of MDA-MB-435-RFP Cells

1. Anesthetize 20 6-week-old female nude mice with the ketamine mixture (described above).

2. Slowly inject MDA-MB-435-RFP cells (5×10^6/100 μl Matrigel) into the mammary fat pad. Press the needle holes in order to prevent any cancer cells overflowing and seeding at the incision site [27].

3.25 Efficacy of S. typhimurium A1-R Administered by Three Different Routes on the Orthotopic MDA-MB-435-RFP Breast Cancer Model (See Note 17)

1. Randomize mice, orthotopically-implanted with MDA-MB-435-RFP, into four groups: Group 1, five mice to serve as untreated controls; group 2, five mice to treat orally (p.o.) with 2×10^8 CFU S. typhimurium A1-R/200 µl, twice a week; group 3, five mice to treat i.v. with 2.5×10^7 CFU S. typhimurium A1-R/100 µl, twice a week; and group 4, five mice to treat i.t. with 2.5×10^7 CFU S. typhimurium A1-R/50 µl, twice per week.

2. Sacrifice the mice on day 34 after treatment.

3. Harvest tumors and homogenize and centrifuge. Plate supernatants on LB medium to detect growth of S. typhimurium A1-R from these tissues.

4. Prepare tissues for standard frozen sectioning and hematoxylin & eosin (H&E) staining for histopathological analysis [27].

3.26 Reversible Skin Flap

1. Make an arc-shaped incision (skin flap) in the skin to image deeper into the tumor tissue. The skin flap can be opened repeatedly to directly image the cancer cells and close simply with a 6-0 suture [28].

2. Anesthetize animals with the ketamine mixture (described above) [11].

3.27 Primer Dose S. typhimurium A1-R Therapy of Lewis Lung Carcinoma (See Note 18)

1. Two weeks after cancer-cell inoculation, treat C57BL/6 mice ($n=5$) bearing subcutaneous LLC tumors expressing RFP (LLC-RFP) with S. typhimurium A1-R (1×10^6 CFU/200 µl PBS) i.v. via the tail vein as a primer dose. Use PBS (i.v.) as a control.

2. Four hours after the primer dose, treat both control and primer dose-treated mice with a high dose of S. typhimurium A1-R (1×10^7 CFU/200 µl PBS). Administer primer dose, or PBS only, followed by a high dose once a week for 4 weeks.

3. Sacrifice mice after 4 weeks administration of bacterial therapy. Remove the tumors and measure their weight [29].

3.28 Effect of S. typhimurium A1-R on TNF-α Induction

1. Use LLC-RFP tumor-bearing C57BL/6 mice for TNF-α determination. Obtain blood samples at various time points after S. typhimurium A1-R dosing.

2. Measure TNF-α with a mouse TNF-α enzyme-linked immunosorbent assay (ELISA) kit [29].

3.29 Orthotopic Pancreatic Cancer Implantation

1. Establish orthotopic human pancreatic cancer xenografts in 6–9-week-old nude mice by SOI of XPA-1-RFP tumor fragments into the tail of the pancreas:

2. After anesthesia, make a small 6–10-mm transverse incision on the left flank of the mouse through the skin and peritoneum. Expose the tail of the pancreas through this incision and suture a single 1 mm³ tumor fragment, harvested from XPA-1-RFP

subcutaneous tumors, on the tail of the pancreas using 8-0 nylon surgical sutures.

3. Upon completion, return the tail of the pancreas to the abdomen and close the incision in one layer using 6-0 nylon surgical sutures [20, 30–34].

3.30 S. typhimurium A1-R Therapy and Chemotherapy on Pancreatic Cancer Stem Cells (See Note 19)

1. Orthotopically implant 6–8-week-old nude mice with each morphological type of XPA-1, spindle (stem cell-like) and round (non-stem cell-like). Treat mice in the following groups: (1) 5-fluorouracil (5-FU) (10 mg/kg, ip), (2) cisplatinum (CDDP) (5 mg/kg, ip), (3) gemcitabine (GEM) (150 mg/kg, ip), (4) *S. typhimurium* A1-R (1.5×10^8 CFU/body, ip), and (5) saline (vehicle/control, ip).

2. Inject chemotherapeutic drugs weekly from day 21 after tumor implantation for 4 weeks. Supply each treatment arm with 8 tumor-bearing mice.

3. Sacrifice animals at 7 weeks and weigh tumors and harvest for analysis.

4. Image GFP and RFP fluorescence using the OV100 imaging or similar system [39] and the FV1000 confocal microscope [23].

3.31 Establishment of Patient-Derived Orthotopic Xenograft (PDOX) Model of Pancreatic Cancer [31]

1. Obtain pancreatic cancer tumor tissue from patients at surgery. Cut the tumor into 1-mm^3 fragments and transplant subcutaneously in NOD/SCID or nude mice (F1 generation) [21, 35, 36]

2. After subcutaneous tumor growth, harvest the tumor, divide the tissue into fragments and transplant to the pancreas using SOI, as described above [31].

3.32 Establishment of Imageable PDOX (iPDOX) Model

1. Using SOI, establish the imageable (iPDOX) model in transgenic RFP or GFP nude mice (F2) [31, 37], from the patient tumor growing in nontransgenic nude mice or other immunodeficient mice.

2. Harvest the tumors from transgenic nude RFP mice and orthotopically passage in non-transgenic nude mice using SOI [21].

3.33 Whole-Body Imaging of iPDOX Model (See Note 20)

1. For whole-body imaging in live mice at variable magnification, use the Olympus OV100 imaging system or equivalent.

2. Process images for contrast and brightness and analyze with the use of Paint Shop Pro 8 and Cell [39].

3.34 Scanning Laser Microscopy of the iPDOX Model

1. Use the Olympus IV100 scanning laser microscope, with a 488 nm argon laser. The novel stick objectives (as small as 1.3 mm) are designed specifically for this laser scanning microscope. The very narrow objectives deliver very high-resolution images.

2. Use a PC computer running FluoView software to control the microscope. Record all images and store as proprietary multilayer 16-bit Tagged Image File Format files [12, 40].

3.35 Orthotopic Implantation of Ovarian Cancer in Nude Mice

1. Establish subcutaneous tumors first by implantation of ovarian cancer cells (5×10^6–1×10^7 in 200-µl Matrigel) in the back skin of female nude mice (5–7 weeks).

2. Anesthetize mice with the ketamine mixture (described above) administered by s.c. injection.

3. For orthotopic implantation, make a right lateral dorsal incision to open the retro-peritoneum and implant one tumor block (2 mm × 2 mm³) on the right ovarian capsule with an 8-0 surgical suture using previously-described methods [41, 42].

4. Close the retro-peritoneum and skin with a 6-0 surgical suture.

3.36 Treatment of Orthotopic Ovarian Cancer [6]

1. Seven days after orthotopic implantation of human SKOV3-GFP ovarian cells as described above, confirm intra-abdominal tumor formation with fluorescence imaging.

2. Divide the mice into three groups:

3. Group 1: Inject i.v. *S. typhimurium* A1-R (5×10^7 CFU) in 100-µl PBS once every 7 days, starting 7 days post-cancer implantation.

4. Group 2: Inject i.p. *S. typhimurium* A1-R (5×10^7 CFU) in 100-µl PBS once every 7 days, starting 7 days after cancer implantation.

5. Group 3: Use a no-treatment group as a control.

6. Determine the overall survival time of each group.

7. Measure the body weight of all mice at day 0, 1, 2, 5, 7, 9, and 14 in order to assess toxicity of *S. typhimurium* A1-R therapy.

3.37 Selection of Breast-Cancer High-Brain-Metastasis Model [9]

1. Use 4T1 murine breast cancer cells expressing RFP.

2. Slowly inject cancer cells, (5.0×10^6/100 µl serum-free medium), into the right second mammary gland underneath the nipple.

3. When the average tumor volume reaches approximately 500–600 mm³, remove the primary tumor on day 14 after tumor implantation.

4. Harvest brain metastases when the mice became moribund.

5. Culture, amplify, and then inject cancer cells from the brain metastasis into the left cardiac ventricle of mice to generate brain metastases again.

6. Repeat for 4 cycles of selection.

7. Anesthetize nude mice i.m. with the ketamine mixture (described above).

8. Inject 4T1-RFP breast cancer cells (1.0×10^6/100 µl serum-free medium) in slowly into the right second mammary gland (underneath the nipple).

9. Press the needle holes in order to prevent any cancer cells overflowing and seeding at the incision site.

10. Resect the primary tumor when the average tumor volume reaches approximately 500–600 mm^3 by day 14 after tumor implantation.

11. Close wounds with 6-0 surgical sutures.

12. Perform all procedures of the operation with a MZ6 ×7 magnification microscope under HEPA-filtered laminar flow hoods.

13. Use the OV100 [39] or IV100 [12], FV1000 [23], or Maestro spectral-separation fluorescence imaging system for imaging [43].

3.38   S. typhimurium A1-R Treatment of Breast-Cancer Brain Metastasis

1. Grow GFP-expressing *S. typhimurium* A1-R overnight in LB medium and then dilute 1:10 in LB medium.

2. Harvest bacteria at late-log phase, wash with PBS, and then dilute in PBS [9].

3. Inject the mice implanted orthotopically with the high-metastatic 4T1 variant i.v. with *S. typhimurium* A1-R (5×10^7 CFU in 100 μl PBS).

4. Identify nude mice with brain metastasis by non-invasive fluorescence imaging 2 weeks after surgical removal of the orthotopic primary tumor.

5. Randomize nude mice into treatment and control groups. Treat mice with *S. typhimurium* A1-R (5×10^7 CFU in 100 μl PBS) via the tail vein once a week for 3 weeks. Compare treated and untreated mice for survival determination for 21 days post-initial treatment.

3.39   Breast-Cancer Experimental Bone-Metastasis Models [10]

1. Harvest MDA-MB-435-GFP cells from subconfluent cell culture plates, wash with PBS, and resuspend in PBS.

2. Anesthetize mice with the ketamine mixture (described above) before injection.

3. Inject cells (2×10^5) into the left cardiac ventricle of female nude mice using a 27-G needle.

4. A successful injection is characterized by the pumping of arterial blood into the syringe.

5. Monitor development of bone metastases with an Illumatool imaging system.

6. Isolate cancer cells from the bone metastasis by sacrifice of the mice and excision of the bone metastasis. Cut open both ends of the bones. Fill a 1-ml syringe with a 27-G needle with PBS and insert into one end of the bone. Force out mouse bone marrow cells as well as cancer cells from the other end of the syringe by applying pressure to the syringe.

7. Collect cells by centrifugation and wash once with PBS before culturing at 37 °C.

8. After 2 weeks of culture, obtain a pure population of human cancer cells as confirmed by fluorescence imaging. Repeat for 4 cycles of this procedure, to obtain a highly metastatic cells line, termed MDA-MB-435-GFP-BM4.

9. Inject MDA-MB-435-GFP-BM4 cells (2×10^5) intracardially in nude mice.

10. Image the mice longitudinally, with the Illumatool or other fluorescence imaging system, after cardiac injection of MDA-MB-435-GFP-BM4 to demonstrate progression of multiple metastases to the skeleton including the skull, femur, and vertebrae.

11. One week after cancer-cell injection, administer *S. typhimurium* A1-R $(5 \times 10^7$ CFU, i.v.) once a week for 3 weeks.

12. Administer the control mice the same volume of PBS.

13. Evaluate metastasis-free survival by non-invasive imaging of the GFP-expressing tumors with the Illumatool instrument or the iBox Scientia Imaging System or equivalent.

14. Define metastasis-free survival as the time from cardiac injection of cancer cells to the time of imaging of bone metastases with the Illumatool or equivalent instrument.

15. At the end of the follow-up, excise the metastases and wash the bone marrow with PBS to confirm the presence of GFP-expressing cancer cells.

16. For an alternative experimental breast-cancer bone-metastasis model, make a midline skin incision (5 mm) just below the knee joint to expose the tibial tuberosity. Co-inject Matrigel (5 µl) and MDA-MB-435-GFP-BM4 cells (5×10^5) into the intramedullary cavity of the tibia with a 0.5-ml 28-G latex-free insulin syringe (0.5 ml 28 G).

17. Close the skin with a 6-0 suture.

18. Two weeks after injection, perform fluorescence imaging to confirm the GFP-expressing tumor is growing, using the iBox or equivalent instrument.

Treatment of Breast-Cancer Experimental Bone-Metastasis Models with S. typhimurium A1-R [10]

1. Administer *S. typhimurium* A1-R $(5 \times 10^7$ CFU, i.v.) to nude mice with bone metastasis once a week for 3 weeks.

2. Administer the same volume of PBS to the remaining mice (untreated control group).

3. Perform fluorescence imaging on treated and untreated mice, and record GFP-expressing fluorescent area every 2 weeks for 12 weeks using the iBox Scientia or equivalent instrument.

3.40 Soft Tissue Sarcoma Model [17]

1. Use 4–6-week-old nude mice.

2. Anesthetize a 6-week-old female nude mice with the ketamine mixture (described above) via s.c. injection.

3. Sterilize the leg with alcohol.

4. Make an approximately 2-mm midline skin incision just above the knee joint to expose the quadriceps femoris muscle.

5. Inject HT-1080-RFP fibrosarcoma cells (1×10^6 per mouse) in Matrigel (5 µl per mouse) into the muscle with a 0.5-ml 28-G latex-free insulin syringe.

6. Close the skin with a 6-0 suture.

7. On day 14 and 21, inject *S. typhimurium* (5×10^7 CFU per mouse) into the tail vein.

8. Sacrifice and perform fluorescence imaging on day 28 to determine the efficacy of bacterial therapy for both primary tumors and lung metastases.

9. Measure the size of the primary tumors (fluorescent area [mm^2]) with the iBox or equivalent instrument.

10. Excise the lung tumor and image the metastases on the surface and count the number of metostasis (*see* **Note 21**) with the OV100 or equivalent instrument.

11. To obtain experimental lung metastasis, inject HT-1080-RFP cells (1×10^6 cells in 100 µl PBS) into the tail vein of nude mice (day 0).

12. On days 7, 14, and 21, inject *S. typhimurium* A1-R (5×10^7 CFU) in the tail vein.

13. On day 28, sacrifice mice and image the lungs to observe lung metastases to determine the efficacy of bacterial therapy. Observe lung metastases in the treated and untreated animals and record the fluorescent areas using the OV100 or equivalent instrument.

4   Notes

1. GFP expression was stable for over 100 passages in *S. typhimurium* A1-R [7].

2. *S. typhimurium* 14028-GFP was treated with nitrosoguanidine (NTG) mutagenesis to obtain auxotrophic mutant bacteria that grew on complete medium, but not minimal medium.

3. Specific auxotrophy was identified by growth in minimal medium supplemented with each amino acid one at a time.

4. Wild-type *S. typhimurium* killed mice within 2 days. The Leu-Arg double-auxotrophic mutant *S. typhimurium* A1 did not

kill mice. Thus, *S. typhimurium* A1 was chosen for initial anti-cancer efficacy studies [7].

5. All observed organs were infected 2–4 days after injection of *S. typhimurium* A1-GFP (1×10^7 CFU per mouse) in nude mice implanted with the human PC-3 prostate cancer. However, GFP-labeled bacteria could not be observed in the spleen, liver, kidney, and lung by day 15. In contrast, the bacteria grew extensively in the implanted PC-3 tumor [7].

6. The enhanced tumor-targeting strain of *S. typhimurium* A1-R was obtained [3] by passage of *S. typhimurium* A1 through HT-29 and HCT-116 human colon tumors growing in nude mice. *S. typhimurium* A1-R was found to have enhanced tumor virulence (please see below).

7. The MARY-X human breast cancer was treated with *S. typhimurium* A1-R in an orthotopic model. Tumor regression occurred following a single i.v. injection of *S. typhimurium* A1-R [27] with four of 10 mice apparent cures [3].

8. Fragmentation of the GFP-expressing nuclei of cancer cells after infection *S. typhimurium* A1 signified apoptosis [7].

9. Lung metastasis was significantly reduced in the *S. typhimurium* A1-R treatment group than control [16].

10. Cancer cells trafficked in the efferent lymph duct toward the axillary lymph node of nude mice immediately after injection [15].

11. All lymph-node metastases had been eradicated by day 7. In contrast, metastases continued to grow in the control group [15].

12. The high-dose bacteria treatment group had significantly less tumor than the un-treated control group demonstrating dose-response [13].

13. *S. typhimurium* A1-R administered i.v. or intrasplenic (i.s.) resulted in lower hepatic and splenic tumor burden compared with untreated control mice [14]. *S. typhimurium* A1-R increased survival time of the treated mice. All results were statistically significant [14].

14. Untreated mice had progressive paralysis beginning at day 6 after tumor transplantation. The untreated mice developed complete paralysis between 18 and 25 days. Mice treated with *S. typhimurium* A1-R i.v. had delayed onset of paralysis. Mice treated with intrathecal administration of *S. typhimurium* A1-R had the longest delay before paralysis. The intrathecally treated mice survived the longest, with less paralysis compared to control or i.v. treated mice [18].

15. Transgenic nestin-driven green fluorescent protein (ND-GFP) mice express GFP in nascent blood vessels. The ear tumor had

more blood vessels as visualized by ND-GFP than the tumor transplanted on the back or footpad. The ear tumor was most sensitive to *i.v.* *S. typhimurium* A1-R due to increased vascularity [12].

16. *S. typhimurium* A1-R administered intracranially (i.c.) inhibited brain-tumor growth approximately eightfold compared with un-treated mice and increased survival by 73 % [19, 44, 45]. Tumors were readily imaged by fluorescence through the cranial window [45].

17. I.v., i.t., and p.o. routes of administration of *S. typhimurium* A1-GFP were compared for targeting of tumor tissue. *S. typhimurium* A1-R-GFP disappeared in normal organs by 2 weeks using each route [27].

18. Immuno-competent mice had a different response to *S. typhimurium* A1-R than immuno-deficient mice. Dosing of *S. typhimurium* A1-R had to be adjusted to avoid toxicity in immuno-competent mice. A primer dose of *S. typhimurium* A1-R was first administered (1×10^6 CFU i.v.) followed by a high dose (1×10^7 CFU i.v.) 4 h later. No side effects were observed with the primer strategy compared to treatment with high-dose alone, where there was toxicity. Tumor vessel destruction was enhanced by primer dosing of *S. typhimurium* A1-R as observed in immuno-competent transgenic mice expressing ND-GFP in nascent blood vessels. Vessel destruction probably increased the anti-tumor efficacy of *S. typhimurium* A1-R [29].

19. The combination *S. typhimurium* A1-R and 5-FU significantly reduced the tumor weight of stem-like (spindle-shaped) and non-stem XPA-1 cells (round). *S. typhimurium* A1-R combined with 5-FU improved antitumor efficacy compared with 5-FU monotherapy on the stem-like spindle XPA-1 cells [46]. 5-FU alone was not active on the stem cells.

20. Light boxes with appropriate filters and camera or even a blue light LED flashlight with an appropriate filter can be used for macro-imaging of GFP-expressing tumors and *S. typhimurium* A1-R-GFP infection [47, 48].

21. *S. typhimurium* A1-R was highly effective against the pancreatic cancer PDOX model [21, 22], ovarian cancer orthotopic model [5, 6] breast cancer brain metastasis model [9], breast cancer bone metastasis model [10] and orthotopic soft-tissue sarcoma model [17].

References

1. Hoffman RM, Zhao M (2014) Methods for the development of tumor-targeting bacteria. Expert Opin Drug Discov 9:741–750
2. Toso JF, Gill VJ, Hwu P, Marincola FM, Restifo NP, Schwartzentruber DJ, Sherry RM et al (2002) Phase I study of the intravenous administration of attenuated Salmonella typhimurium to patients with metastatic melanoma. J Clin Oncol 20:142–152
3. Zhao M, Yang M, Ma H, Li X, Tan X, Li S et al (2006) Targeted therapy with a Salmonella typhimurium leucine-arginine auxotroph cures orthotopic human breast tumors in nude mice. Cancer Res 66:7647–7652
4. Zhang Y, Zhang N, Zhao M, Hoffman RM (2015) Comparison of the selective targeting of Salmonella typhimurium A1-R and VNP20009 on the Lewis lung carcinoma in nude mice. Oncotarget 6:14625–14631
5. Matsumoto Y, Miwa S, Zhang Y, Hiroshima Y, Yano S, Uehara F et al (2014) Efficacy of tumor-targeting Salmonella typhimurium A1-R on nude mouse models of metastatic and disseminated human ovarian cancer. J Cell Biochem 115:1996–2003
6. Matsumoto Y, Miwa S, Zhang Y, Zhao M, Yano S, Uehara F et al (2015) Intraperitoneal administration of tumor-targeting Salmonella typhimurium A1-R inhibits disseminated human ovarian cancer and extends survival in nude mice. Oncotarget 6:11369–11377
7. Zhao M, Yang M, Li X-M, Jiang P, Baranov E, Li S et al (2005) Tumor-targeting bacterial therapy with amino acid auxotrophs of GFP-expressing Salmonella typhimurium. Proc Natl Acad Sci U S A 102:755–760
8. Zhao M, Geller J, Ma H, Yang M, Penman S, Hoffman RM (2007) Monotherapy with a tumor-targeting mutant of Salmonella typhimurium cures orthotopic metastatic mouse models of human prostate cancer. Proc Natl Acad Sci U S A 104:10170–10174
9. Zhang Y, Miwa S, Zhang N, Hoffman RM, Zhao M (2015) Tumor-targeting Salmonella typhimurium A1-R arrests growth of breast-cancer brain metastasis. Oncotarget 6:2615–2622
10. Miwa S, Yano S, Zhang Y, Matsumoto Y, Uehara F, Yamamoto M et al (2014) Tumor-targeting Salmonella typhimurium A1-R prevents experimental human breast cancer bone metastasis in nude mice. Oncotarget 5:7119–7125
11. Uchugonova A, Zhao M, Zhang Y, Weinigel M, König K, Hoffman RM (2012) Cancer-cell killing by engineered Salmonella imaged by multiphoton tomography in live mice. Anticancer Res 32:4331–4337
12. Liu F, Zhang L, Hoffman RM, Zhao M (2010) Vessel destruction by tumor-targeting Salmonella typhimurium A1-R is enhanced by high tumor vascularity. Cell Cycle 9:4518–4524
13. Nagakura C, Hayashi K, Zhao M, Yamauchi K, Yamamoto N, Tsuchiya H et al (2009) Efficacy of a genetically-modified Salmonella typhimurium in an orthotopic human pancreatic cancer in nude mice. Anticancer Res 29:1873–1878
14. Yam C, Zhao M, Hayashi K, Ma H, Kishimoto H, McElroy M et al (2010) Monotherapy with a tumor-targeting mutant of Salmonella typhimurium inhibits liver metastasis in a mouse model of pancreatic cancer. J Surg Res 164:248–255
15. Hayashi K, Zhao M, Yamauchi K, Yamamoto N, Tsuchiya H, Tomita K et al (2009) Cancer metastasis directly eradicated by targeted therapy with a modified Salmonella typhimurium. J Cell Biochem 106:992–998
16. Hayashi K, Zhao M, Yamauchi K, Yamamoto N, Tsuchiya H, Tomita K et al (2009) Systemic targeting of primary bone tumor and lung metastasis of high-grade osteosarcoma in nude mice with a tumor-selective strain of Salmonella typhimurium. Cell Cycle 8:870–875
17. Miwa S, Zhang Y, Baek K-E, Uehara F, Yano S, Yamamoto M et al (2014) Inhibition of spontaneous and experimental lung metastasis of soft-tissue sarcoma by tumor-targeting Salmonella typhimurium A1-R. Oncotarget 5:12849–12861
18. Kimura H, Zhang L, Zhao M, Hayashi K, Tsuchiya H, Tomita K et al (2010) Targeted therapy of spinal cord glioma with a genetically-modified Salmonella typhimurium. Cell Prolif 43:41–48
19. Momiyama M, Zhao M, Kimura H, Tran B, Chishima T, Bouvet M et al (2012) Inhibition and eradication of human glioma with tumor-targeting Salmonella typhimurium in an orthotopic nude-mouse model. Cell Cycle 11:628–632
20. Hiroshima Y, Zhao M, Zhang Y, Maawy A, Hassanein MK, Uehara F et al (2013) Comparison of efficacy of Salmonella typhimurium A1-R and chemotherapy on stem-like and non-stem human pancreatic cancer cells. Cell Cycle 12:2774–2780
21. Hiroshima Y, Zhao M, Maawy A, Zhang Y, Katz MH, Fleming JB et al (2014) Efficacy of Salmonella typhimurium A1-R versus

chemotherapy on a pancreatic cancer patient-derived orthotopic xenograft (PDOX). J Cell Biochem 115:1254–1261

22. Hiroshima Y, Zhang Y, Murakami T, Maawy A, Miwa S, Yamamoto M (2014) Efficacy of tumor-targeting Salmonella typhimurium A1-R in combination with anti-angiogenesis therapy on a pancreatic cancer patient-derived orthotopic xenograft (PDOX) and cell-line mouse models. Oncotarget 5:12346–12356

23. Uchugonova A, Duong J, Zhang N, König K, Hoffman RM (2011) The bulge area is the origin of nestin-expressing pluripotent stem cells of the hair follicle. J Cell Biochem 112:2046–2050

24. Zhao M, Suetsugu A, Ma H, Zhang L, Liu F, Zhang Y et al (2012) Efficacy against lung metastasis with a tumor-targeting mutant of Salmonella typhimurium in immunocompetent mice. Cell Cycle 11:187–193

25. Alpaugh ML, Tomlinson JS, Ye Y, Barsky SH (2002) Relationship of sialyl-Lewis[x/a] underexpression and E-cadherin overexpression in the lymphovascular embolus of inflammatory breast carcinoma. Am J Pathol 161:619–628

26. Basso DM, Beattie MS, Bresnahan JC, Anderson DK, Faden AI, Gruner JA et al (1996) MASCIS evaluation of open field locomotor scores: effects of experience and teamwork on reliability. Multicenter Animal Spinal Cord Injury Study. J Neurotrauma 13:343–359

27. Zhang Y, Tome Y, Suetsugu A, Zhang L, Zhang N, Hoffman RM et al (2012) Determination of the optimal route of administration of Salmonella typhimurium A1-R to target breast cancer in nude mice. Anticancer Res 32:2501–2508

28. Yang M, Baranov E, Wang J-W, Jiang P, Wang X, Sun F-X et al (2002) Direct external imaging of nascent cancer, tumor progression, angiogenesis, and metastasis on internal organs in the fluorescent orthotopic model. Proc Natl Acad Sci U S A 99:3824–3829

29. Tome Y, Zhang Y, Momiyama M, Maehara H, Kanaya F, Tomita K et al (2013) Primer dosing of S. typhimurium A1-R potentiates tumor-targeting and efficacy in immunocompetent mice. Anticancer Res 33:97–102

30. Furukawa T, Kubota T, Watanabe M, Kitajima M, Hoffman RM (1993) A novel "patient-like" treatment model of human pancreatic cancer constructed using orthotopic transplantation of histologically intact human tumor tissue in nude mice. Cancer Res 53:3070–3072

31. Fu X, Guadagni F, Hoffman RM (1992) A metastatic nude mouse model of human pancreatic cancer constructed orthotopically with histologically intact patient specimens. Proc Natl Acad Sci U S A 89:5645–5649

32. Hoffman RM (1999) Orthotopic metastatic mouse models for anticancer drug discovery and evaluation: a bridge to the clinic. Invest New Drugs 17:343–359

33. Bouvet M, Wang J-W, Nardin SR, Nassirpour R, Yang M, Baranov E et al (2002) Real-time optical imaging of primary tumor growth and multiple metastatic events in a pancreatic cancer orthotopic model. Cancer Res 62:1534–1540

34. Bouvet M, Yang M, Nardin S, Wang X, Jiang P, Baranov E et al (2000) Chronologically-specific metastatic targeting of human pancreatic tumors in orthotopic models. Clin Exp Metastasis 18:213–218

35. Kim MP, Evans DB, Wang H, Abbruzzese JL, Fleming JB, Gallick GE (2009) Generation of orthotopic and heterotopic human pancreatic cancer xenografts in immunodeficient mice. Nat Protoc 4:1670–1680

36. Kim MP, Truty MJ, Choi W, Kang Y, Chopin-Lally X, Gallick GE et al (2012) Molecular profiling of direct xenograft tumors established from human pancreatic adenocarcinoma after neoadjuvant therapy. Ann Surg Oncol 19(Suppl3):S395–S403

37. Yang M, Reynoso J, Bouvet M, Hoffman RM (2009) A transgenic red fluorescent protein-expressing nude mouse for color-coded imaging of the tumor microenvironment. J Cell Biochem 106:279–284

38. Katz M, Takimoto S, Spivack D, Moossa AR, Hoffman RM, Bouvet M (2003) A novel red fluorescent protein orthotopic pancreatic cancer model for the preclinical evaluation of chemotherapeutics. J Surg Res 113:151–160

39. Yamauchi K, Yang M, Jiang P, Xu M, Yamamoto N, Tsuchiya H et al (2006) Development of real-time subcellular dynamic multicolor imaging of cancer-cell trafficking in live mice with a variable-magnification whole-mouse imaging system. Cancer Res 66:4208–4214

40. Yang M, Jiang P, Hoffman RM (2007) Whole-body subcellular multicolor imaging of tumor-host interaction and drug response in real time. Cancer Res 67:5195–5200

41. Fu X, Hoffman RM (1993) Human ovarian carcinoma metastatic models constructed in nude mice by orthotopic transplantation of histologically-intact patient specimens. Anticancer Res 13:283–286

42. Kiguchi K, Kubota T, Aoki D, Udagawa Y, Yamanouchi S, Saga M et al (1998) A patient-like orthotopic implantation nude mouse model of highly metastatic human ovarian cancer. Clin Exp Metastasis 16:751–756

43. Zhang Y, Hiroshima Y, Ma H, Zhang N, Zhao M, Hoffman RM (2015) Complementarity of variable-magnification and spectral-separation fluorescence imaging systems for noninvasive detection of metastasis and intravital detection of single cancer cells in mouse models. Anticancer Res 35:661–667

44. Momiyama M, Suetsugu A, Chishima T, Bouvet M, Endo I, Hoffman RM (2013) Subcellular real-time imaging of the efficacy of temozolomide on cancer cells in the brain of live mice. Anticancer Res 33:103–106

45. Momiyama M, Suetsugu A, Kimura H, Chishima T, Bouvet M, Endo I et al (2013) Dynamic subcellular imaging of cancer cell mitosis in the brain of live mice. Anticancer Res 33:1367–1371

46. Hassanein MK, Suetsugu A, Saji S, Moriwaki H, Bouvet M, Moossa AR et al (2011) Stem-like and non-stem human pancreatic cancer cells distinguished by morphology and metastatic behavior. J Cell Biochem 112:3549–3554

47. Hoffman RM, Zhao M (2006) Whole-body imaging of bacterial infection and antibiotic response. Nat Protoc 1:2988–2994

48. Yang M, Luiken G, Baranov E, Hoffman RM (2005) Facile whole-body imaging of internal fluorescent tumors in mice with an LED flashlight. Biotechniques 39:170–172

Chapter 14

Salmonella typhimurium A1-R and Cell-Cycle Decoy Therapy of Cancer

Robert M. Hoffman and Shuya Yano

Abstract

Cancer cells in G_0/G_1 are resistant to cytotoxic chemotherapy agents which kill only cycling cancer cells. *Salmonella typhimurium* A1-R (*S. typhimurium* A1-R) decoyed cancer cells in monolayer culture and in tumor spheres to cycle from G_0/G_1 to $S/G_2/M$, as demonstrated by fluorescence ubiquitination-based cell cycle indicator (FUCCI) imaging. *S. typhimurium* A1-R targeted FUCCI-expressing subcutaneous tumors, and tumors growing on the liver, growing in nude mice and also decoyed quiescent cancer cells, which were the majority of the cells in the tumors, to cycle from G_0/G_1 to $S/G_2/M$. The *S. typhimurium* A1-R-decoyed cancer cells became sensitive to cytotoxic agents.

Key words *Salmonella typhimurium* A1-R, Tumor-targeting, Cell cycle, Decoy, Amino acid, Auxotroph, Chemotherapy, Fluorescence ubiquitination-based cell cycle indicator (FUCCI), Imaging, Green fluorescent protein (GFP)Red fluorescent protein (RFP), Surgical orthotopic implantation (SOI), Nude mice, Mouse models, Cancer, Metastasis

1 Introduction

Drug resistance in cancer is the major problem in cancer therapy. Using a fluorescence ubiquitination cell cycle indicator (FUCCI), we determined that approximately 80 % of total cells of an established tumor are in G_0/G_1 phase and thereby resistant to cytotoxic drugs. Cytotoxic agents killed only proliferating cancer cells at the surface and, in contrast, had little effect on quiescent cancer cells. Moreover, resistant quiescent cancer cells restarted cycling after the cessation of chemotherapy demonstrating a probable major basis for resistance of solid tumors to chemotherapy [1] (Figs. 1, 2, 3, 4, and 5).

As described in this chapter, we subsequently observed that *S. typhimurium* A1-R decoyed cancer cells in tumors, to cycle from G_0/G_1 to $S/G_2/M$, thereby making them sensitive to cytotoxic agents [2] (Figs. 6, 7, 8, and 9).

Robert M. Hoffman (ed.), *Bacterial Therapy of Cancer: Methods and Protocols*, Methods in Molecular Biology, vol. 1409, DOI 10.1007/978-1-4939-3515-4_14, © Springer Science+Business Media New York 2016

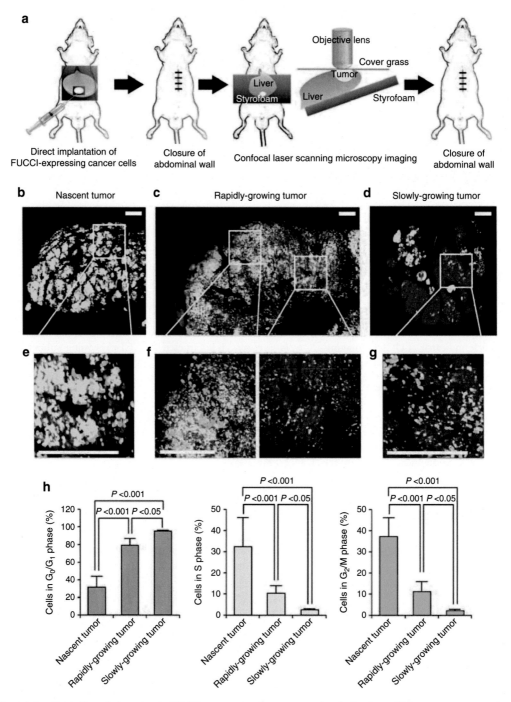

Fig. 1 Intravital cell-cycle imaging in FUCCI-expressing tumors growing in the liver. All images were acquired with the FV1000 (Olympus) confocal laser scanning microscope (CLSM). The FUCCI-expressing cancer cells in G_0/G_1, S, or G_2/M phases appear *red*, *yellow*, or *green*, respectively. (**a**) Schematic diagram shows the method of repeated intravital CLSM imaging of FUCCI-expressing gastric cancer cells growing in the liver. (**b–d**) Representative images of FUCCI-expressing tumors in the liver of live mice. Nascent tumor 7 days after implantation (**b**); rapidly growing tumor 90 days after implantation (**c**); slowly growing tumor 90 days after implantation (**d**). (**e–g**) High-magnification images of FUCCI-expressing cancer cells are shown. (**h**) Bar graphs show the distribution of FUCCI-expressing cells in a nascent tumor, a rapidly growing tumor, and a slowly growing tumor. Data are means ± SD (each group for $n = 10$). Scale bars represent 500 μm [1]

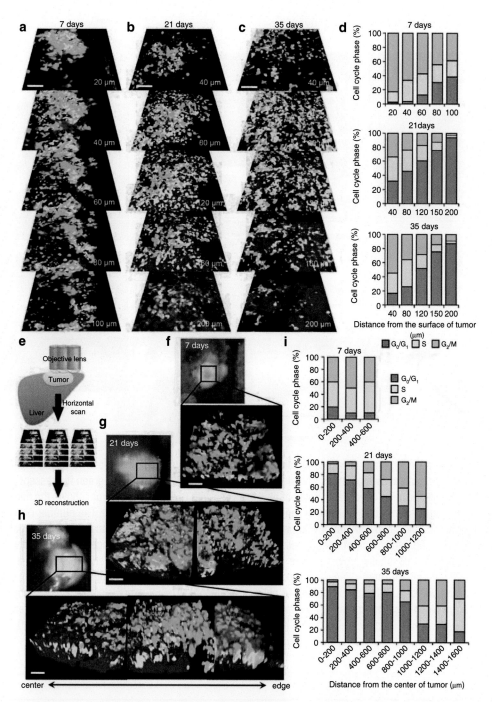

Fig. 2 Cell-cycle-phase distribution of cancer cells at the tumor surface and center. (**a–c**) FUCCI-expressing MKN45 stomach cancer cells were implanted directly in the liver of nude mice and imaged at 7 days (**a**), 21 days (**b**), or 35 days (**c**). (**d**) Histograms show the cell-cycle distribution in the tumor at 7 days (*top*), 21 days (*middle*), and 35 days (*lower*) after implantation. (**e**) Schematic diagram of in vivo CLSM imaging of different-sized tumors. Tumors were scanned from the center to the edge. The scanned images were then three-dimensionally reconstructed. (**f–h**) Representative 3D reconstruction images of a nascent tumor at 7 days after cancer-cell implantation (**f**), 21 days (**g**), and 35 days (**h**) after implantation. (**i**) Histograms show the distribution of FUCCI-expressing cells at different distances from the center. The number of cells in each cell-cycle phase was assessed by counting the number of cells of each color at the indicated time points and depth. The percentages of cells in the G_2/M, S, and G_0/G_1 phases of the cell cycle are shown (**e** and **i**). Data are means (each group for $n = 5$). Scale bars represent 100 μm [1]

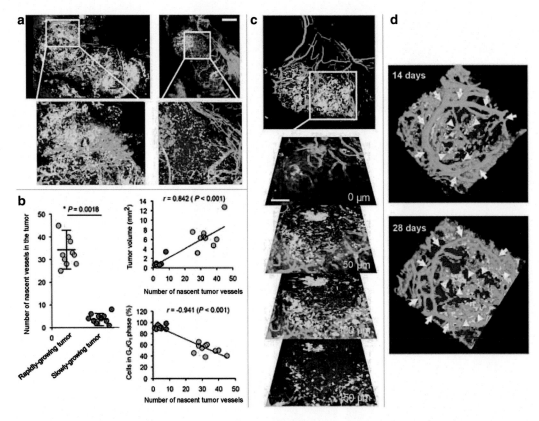

Fig. 3 Imaging nascent tumor vessels and cancer cell-cycle phase in rapidly and slowly growing tumors. (**a**) Comparison of rapidly-growing tumors and slowly-growing tumors in nestin-driven green fluorescent protein (ND-GFP) transgenic mice, which label nascent blood vessels with GFP. (**b**) Scatter-gram shows the number of GFP-expressing nascent tumor vessels in rapidly- and slowly-growing tumors (*left*). The number of nascent tumor vessels is associated with tumor volume (*upper right*). The number of nascent tumor vessels negatively-correlates with the percentage of cancer cells in G_0/G_1 phase (*lower right*). (**c**) Images of FUCCI-expressing cancer cells in a large rapidly-growing tumor in the liver at 28 days after implantation are shown at different depths in the tumor. (**d**) Three-dimensional reconstruction of a tumor at 14 days (*upper*) and 28 days (*lower*) after implantation of FUCCI-expressing MKN45 cells in the liver of ND-GFP-expressing transgenic nude mice. Fine nascent blood vessels expressing GFP are indicated with *arrowheads*, and the trunk of blood vessels is indicated with *arrows*. Data are means (each group for $n=5$). Scale bars represent (**a**) 500 μm; (**c**) 100 μm [1]

Fig. 4 Spatial–temporal response to cytotoxic chemotherapy of cells in various phases of the cell cycle in tumors. (**a**) A schematic diagram showing longitudinal CSLM imaging of an FUCCI-expressing tumor after chemotherapy. (**b**) Representative image of an FUCCI-expressing tumor in the liver before and after cisplatinum (CDDP) treatment. (**c**) Images of FUCCI-expressing cancer cells are shown at different depths in the tumor at indicated time points noted in **b**. (**d**) Representative images of an FUCCI-expressing tumor in the liver before and after paclitaxel treatment. (**e**) Images of FUCCI-expressing cancer cells are shown at different depths in the tumor at indicated time points noted in **d**. (**f**) Histograms show the cell-cycle-phase distribution of cancer cells in the tumor at indicated time points. Data are means ± SD (each group for $n=5$). Scale bars represent 500 μm [1]

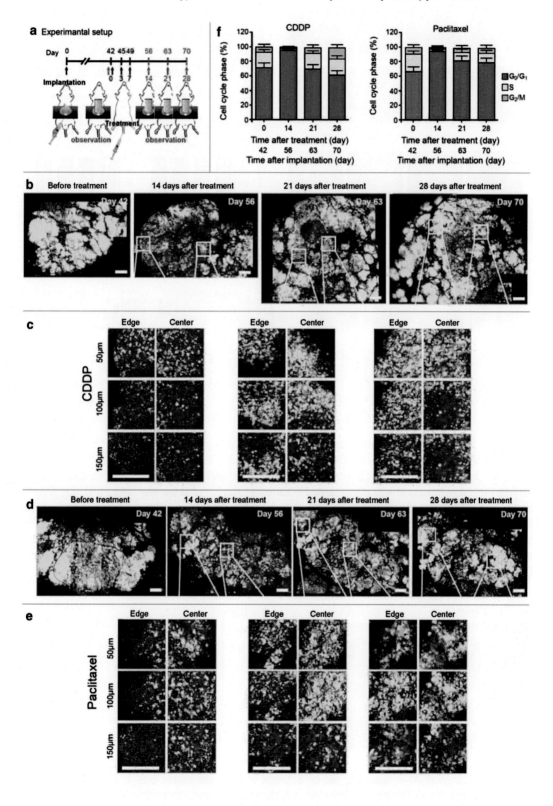

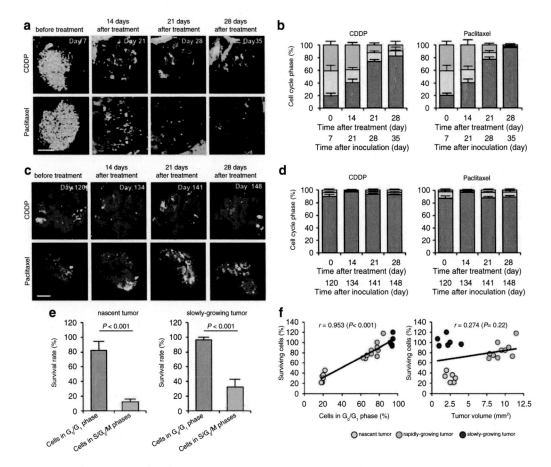

Fig. 5 The efficacy of chemotherapy depends on the cell-cycle-phase distribution within the tumor. (**a**) Representative images of nascent FUCCI-expressing tumor in the liver before and after CDDP or paclitaxel treatment. (**b**) Histograms show the cell-cycle-phase distribution within the tumor at the indicated time points. (**c**) Representative images of a slowly-growing FUCCI-expressing tumor in the liver before and after CDDP or paclitaxel treatment. (**d**) Histograms show the cell-cycle-phase distribution within the tumor at the indicated time points. (**e**) Histograms show the survival rate of the cancer cells in G_0/G_1 phase or in $S/G_2/M$ phase after chemotherapy. (**f**) Relationship between the percentage of cells in G_0/G_1 phases before treatment and surviving-cell fraction (*left*). Relationship between tumor size before treatment and surviving-cell fraction (*right*). Data are means ± SD (each group for $n = 3$). Scale bars = 500 μm [1]

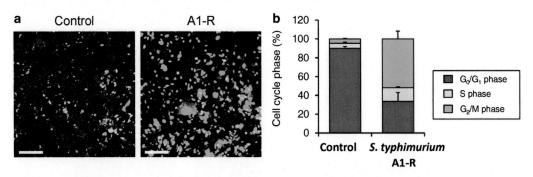

Fig. 6 *S. typhimurium* A1-R stimulates cell-cycle transit of quiescent cancer cells in monolayer culture. *S. typhimurium* A1-R targeted quiescent cancer cells and stimulated cell-cycle transit from G_0/G_1 to $S/G_2/M$ phases. (**a**) Representative images of control cancer cells and cancer cells treated with *S. typhimurium* A1-R. (**b**) Histograms show cell-cycle distribution in control and *S. typhimurium* A1-R-treated cultures. Scale bar: 500 μm [2]

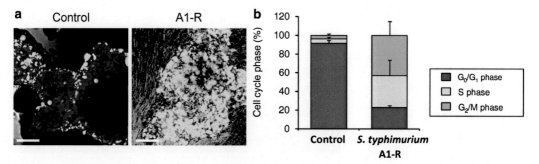

Fig. 7 *S. typhimurium* A1-R stimulates cell-cycle transit in quiescent tumor spheres in vitro. *S. typhimurium* A1-R stimulated cell-cycle transit from G_0/G_1 to $S/G_2/M$ phases. (**a**) Representative images of control tumor spheres and tumor spheres treated with *S. typhimurium* A1-R. (**b**) Histograms show cell-cycle distribution in control and *S. typhimurium* A1-R-treated tumor spheres. Scale bar: 500 µm [2]

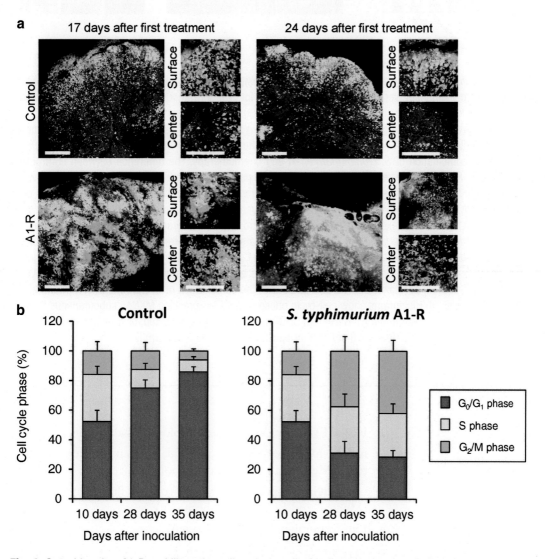

Fig. 8 *S. typhimurium* A1-R mobilizes the cell-cycle transit of quiescent cancer cells in tumors in vivo. (**a**) Representative images of cross sections of FUCCI-expressing MKN45 tumor xenografts treated with *S. typhimurium* A1-R or untreated control. (**b**) Histograms show the cell-cycle-phase distribution of FUCCI-expressing cells within the tumor treated with *S. typhimurium* A1-R or untreated control. Scale bars: 500 µm [2]

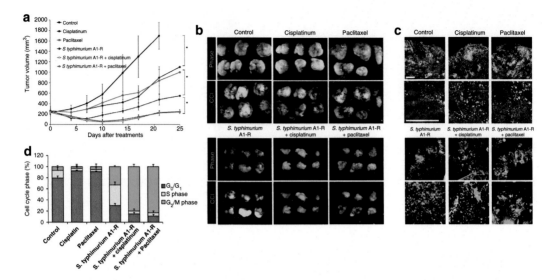

Fig. 9 *S. typhimurium* A1-R-decoyed tumors became sensitive to chemotherapy. FUCCI-expressing MKN45 cells (5×10^6 cells/mouse) were injected subcutaneously into the left flank of nude mice. When the tumors reached approximately 8 mm in diameter (tumor volume, 300 mm³), mice were administered iv *S. typhimurium* A1-R alone, or with CDDP (4 mg/kg ip) or paclitaxel (5 mg/kg ip) for five cycles every 3 days. (**a**) Growth curves of tumors derived from FUCCI-expressing MKN45 cells after treatment with chemotherapy, *S. typhimurium* A1-R, or the combination of *S. typhimurium* A1-R and chemotherapy. The difference between control and CDDP treated: $P < 0.01$; the difference between control and paclitaxel treated: $P < 0.05$; the difference between control and *S. typhimurium* A1-R-treated: $P < 0.05$; the difference between control and the combination of *S. typhimurium* A1-R and CDDP-treated: $P < 0.01$; the difference between control and the combination of *S. typhimurium* A1-R and paclitaxel-treated: $P < 0.01$. (**b**) Macroscopic photographs of FUCCI-expressing tumors: untreated control; *S. typhimurium* A1-R treated; CDDP-treated; paclitaxel-treated; or treated with the combination of *S. typhimurium* A1-R and either CDDP or paclitaxel. Scale bars: 10 mm. (**c**) Representative images of cross sections of FUCCI-expressing MKN45 subcutaneous tumors: untreated control; *S. typhimurium* A1-R-treated; CDDP-treated; paclitaxel-treated; or treated with the combination of *S. typhimurium* A1-R and either CDDP or paclitaxel. (**d**) Histograms show cell-cycle phase of FUCCI-expressing MKN45 subcutaneous tumors: untreated control; *S. typhimurium* A1-R treated; CDDP-treated; paclitaxel-treated; or treated with the combination of *S. typhimurium* A1-R and either CDDP or paclitaxel. Scale bars: 500 μm [2]

2   Materials

1. FUCCI vectors (Medical and Biological Laboratory).

2. mKO2-hCdt1-expressing plasmids (green fluorescent protein) (Medical and Biological Laboratory).

3. mAG-hGem-expressing plasmids (orange fluorescent protein) (Medical and Biological Laboratory).

4. Lipofectamine™ LTX (Invitrogen).

5. Trypsin-EDTA (Fisher Scientific).

6. 96-well plates (Fisher Scientific).

7. LB medium (Fisher Scientific).

8. FACSAria cell sorter (Becton Dickinson).

9. MKN45 stomach adenocarcinoma cell line (Okayama University).

10. Athymic nu/nu nude mice (AntiCancer Inc.).

11. Autoclaved laboratory rodent diet (Teklad LM-485; Harlan).

12. Ketamine mixture (10 μl ketamine HCl, 7.6 μl xylazine, 2.4 μl acepromazine maleate, and 10 μl PBS) (Henry-Schein).

13. *S. typhimurium* A1-R (AntiCancer Inc.).

14. Cisplatinum (Pharmaceutical Buyers International).

15. Paclitaxel (Pharmaceutical Buyers International).

16. FV1000 (Olympus).

3 Methods

3.1 FUCCI

1. Generate the FUCCI probe by fusing mKO2 (monomeric kusabira orange2) and mAG (monomeric azami green) to the ubiquitination domains of human Cdt1 and geminin, respectively.

2. Transfect plasmids expressing mKO2-hCdt1 into MKN45 cells using Lipofectamine™ LTX.

3. Incubate the cells for 48 h after transfection and then trypsinize and seed in 96-well plates at a density of 10 cells/well.

4. In the first step, sort S-, G_2-,, and M-phase cells using a FACSAria cell sorter or equivalent.

5. Re-transfect the first-step-sorted green fluorescent cells with mAG-hGem (orange) and then sort for orange fluorescence [2, 3].

3.2 Cells

1. Use the radio-resistant poorly differentiated stomach adenocarcinoma cell line, MKN45, which is derived from a liver metastasis of a patient or other cancer cell lines [2, 3].

3.3 Animal Experiments

1. Maintain the athymic nu/nu nude mice in a barrier facility under HEPA filtration and feed mice with an autoclaved laboratory rodent diet.

2. Conduct all animal studies in accordance with the principles and procedures outlined in the National Institute of Health Guide for the Care and Use of Animals [2].

3.4 Tumor Model

1. Harvest FUCCI-expressing MKN45 cells from monolayer culture by brief trypsinization.

2. Prepare single-cell suspensions at a final concentration of 5×10^6 cells and inject subcutaneously in the left flank of nude mice [2].

3. Perform all animal procedures under anesthesia using s.c. administration of a ketamine mixture (10 μl ketamine HCl, 7.6 μl xylazine, 2.4 μl acepromazine maleate, and 10 μl PBS).

3.5 Growth of S. typhimurium A1-R

1. Grow GFP-expressing *S. typhimurium* A1-R bacteria overnight in LB medium and then dilute 1:10 in LB medium.

2. Harvest bacteria at late-log phase, wash with PBS, and then dilute in PBS [4].

3.6 Decoy Chemotherapy (See Notes 1–4)

1. When the tumors reach approximately 8 mm in diameter (tumor volume, 300 mm³), administer the mice *S. typhimurium* A1-R iv, alone or in combination with cisplatinum (4 mg/kg ip) or paclitaxel (5 mg/kg ip) for five cycles every 3 days [2].

4 Notes

1. S. typhimurium A1-R stimulates cell-cycle transit of quiescent cancer cells in monolayer culture: Time-lapse imaging of *S. typhimurium* A1-R interacting with quiescent FUCCI-expressing MKN45 cancer cells in monolayer culture demonstrated that *S. typhimurium* A1-R targets quiescent cancer cells and induces their cell-cycle transit from G_0/G_1 to $S/G_2/M$ phase (Fig. 6) [2].

2. S. typhimurium A1-R stimulates cell-cycle transit in quiescent tumor spheres: *S. typhimurium* A1-R targeted quiescent tumor spheres and stimulated cell-cycle transit, of the cancer cells within the spheres, from G_0/G_1 to $S/G_2/M$ phases (Fig. 7) [2].

3. S. typhimurium A1-R mobilizes the cell-cycle transit of quiescent cancer cells in tumors in vivo: Before *S. typhimurium* A1-R treatment, FUCCI-expressing MKN45 tumors had approximately 95 % of the cancer cells in G_0/G_1 after 35 days' growth in nude mice. Thirty-five days after treatment with *S. typhimurium* A1-R, approximately 30 % of the cancer cells were in G_0/G_1 and 70 % in $S/G_2/M$ (Fig. 8) [2].

4. S. typhimurium-decoyed tumors became sensitive to chemotherapy: *S. typhimurium* A1-R sensitized the tumors to chemotherapy due to cell-cycle decoy of the cancer cells within the tumor (Fig. 9) [2].

FUCCI imaging demonstrated that the combination of *S. typhimurium* A1-R cell-cycle decoy and chemotherapy can effectively kill quiescent cancer cells that are resistant to conventional chemotherapy, including in cancer cells and tumors in vivo. The combination of *S. typhimurium* A1-R and either cisplatinum or paclitaxel was highly effective [2].

We previously demonstrated with FUCCI imaging that cancer cells in G_0/G_1 phase can migrate faster and further than cancer cells in $S/G_2/M$ phases. When cancer cells in G_0/G_1 cycled into $S/G_2/M$ phases, they ceased movement and then only restarted migration after reentry into G_0/G_1 phase after cell division. Chemotherapy had little effect on G_0/G_1-invading cancer cells. *S. typhimurium* A1-R decoy chemotherapy may also be useful to target invasive cancer cells, which may otherwise be highly chemo-resistant [2, 5].

References

1. Yano S, Zhang Y, Miwa S, Tome Y, Hiroshima Y, Uehara F et al (2014) Spatial-temporal FUCCI imaging of each cell in a tumor demonstrates locational dependence of cell cycle dynamics and chemoresponsiveness. Cell Cycle 13:2110–2119
2. Yano S, Zhang Y, Zhao M, Hiroshima Y, Miwa S, Uehara F et al (2014) Tumor-targeting *Salmonella typhimurium* A1-R decoys quiescent cancer cells to cycle as visualized by FUCCI imaging and become sensitive to chemotherapy. Cell Cycle 13:3958–3963
3. Yano S, Tazawa H, Hashimoto Y, Shirakawa Y, Kuroda S, Nishizaki M et al (2013) A genetically engineered oncolytic adenovirus decoys and lethally traps quiescent cancer stem-like cells into $S/G_2/M$ phases. Clin Cancer Res 19:6495–6505
4. Miwa S, Yano S, Zhang Y, Matsumoto Y, Uehara F, Yamamoto M et al (2014) Tumor-targeting *Salmonella typhimurium* A1-R prevents experimental human breast cancer bone metastasis in nude mice. Oncotarget 5:7119–7125
5. Yano S, Miwa S, Mii S, Hiroshima Y, Uehara F, Yamamoto M et al (2014) Invading cancer cells are predominantly in G_0/G_1 resulting in chemoresistance demonstrated by real-time FUCCI imaging. Cell Cycle 13:953–960

Chapter 15

Future of Bacterial Therapy of Cancer

Robert M. Hoffman

Abstract

Bacterial therapy of cancer has a centuries-long history and was first-line therapy at the hospital in New York City that would become Memorial Sloan-Kettering Cancer Center, under Dr. William B. Coley. However, after Coley's death in 1936, bacterial therapy of cancer ceased in the clinic until the present century. Clinical trials have been recently carried out for strains of the obligate anaerobe *Clostridium novyi* with the toxin gene deleted, and on an attenuated strain of *Salmonella typhimurium* (*S. typhimurium*), which is a facultative anaerobe that can grow in viable, as well as necrotic, areas of tumors, unlike *Clostridium*, which can only grow in the hypoxic areas. Our laboratory has developed the novel strain *S. typhimurium* A1-R that is effective against all tumor types in clinically-relevant mouse models, including patient-derived orthotopic xenograft (PDOX) mouse models. This chapter suggests future clinical applications for *S. typhimurium* A1-R.

Key words *Salmonella typhimurium* A1-R, Tumor-targeting, Cell cycle, Decoy, Amino acid, Auxotroph, Combination chemotherapy, Fluorescence ubiquitination-based cell cycle indicator (FUCCI), Imaging, Green fluorescent protein (GFP), Surgical orthotopic implantation (SOI), Nude mice, Mouse models, Cancer, Metastasis, Orthotopic

1 Mode of Killing Cancer Cells by Bacteria

The future success of bacterial therapy of cancer depends in part how bacteria kill different types of cancer cells.

To further understand the tumor-killing mechanism of *S. typhimurium* A1-R, we have studied the interaction of *S. typhimurium* A1-R-GFP with three different prostate cancer cell lines in vitro visualized by confocal fluorescence microscopy. We found that *S. typhimurium* A1-R induced cancer cell death by different mechanisms in different cancer cell lines with apoptosis and necrosis in the human PC-3 prostate cancer cell line, and by cell bursting in the human LNCaP and DU-145 prostate cancer cell lines. The time for *S. typhimurium* A1-R-GFP to kill the majority of the cancer cells varied from line to line, ranging from 2 to 48 h (Figs. 1, 2 and 3) [1].

Robert M. Hoffman (ed.), *Bacterial Therapy of Cancer: Methods and Protocols*, Methods in Molecular Biology, vol. 1409, DOI 10.1007/978-1-4939-3515-4_15, © Springer Science+Business Media New York 2016

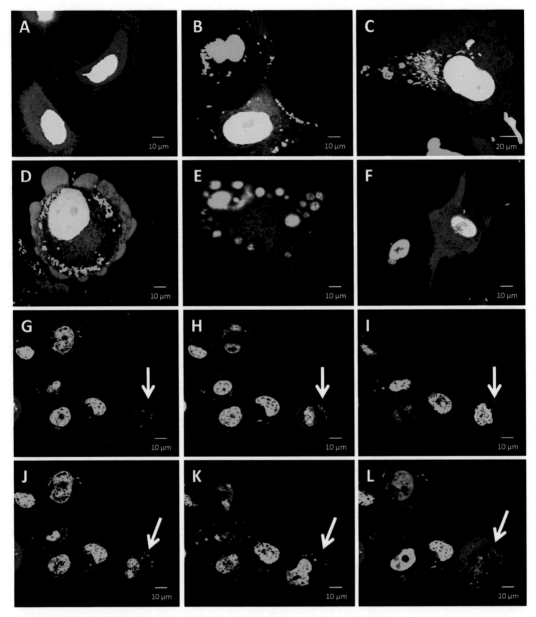

Fig. 1 Dual-color PC-3 human prostate cancer cell death induced by *S. typhimurium* A1-R-GFP. (**a**) Untreated dual-color PC-3 human prostate cancer cells with GFP expressed in the nuclei and RFP expressed in the cytoplasm (0 time point); (**b**) *S. typhimurium* A1-R-GFP attached to the membrane of PC-3 cells (45-min time point); (**c**) *S. typhimurium* A1-R-GFP invasion and proliferation in PC-3 cells (45-min time point); (**d**) cytoplasm swelling in PC-3 cells induced by *S. typhimurium* A1-R-GFP (2-h time point); (**e, f**) apoptotic bodies in PC-3 cells induced by *S. typhimurium* A1-R-GFP invasion (2-h time point); (**g–l**) PC-3 necrotic cell death (*white arrows*) induced by *S. typhimurium* A1-R-GFP invasion (**g** = 45-min time point; **h** = 55-min time point; **i** = 65-min time point; **j** = 1 h, 15-min time point; **k** = 1 h, 25-min time point; **l** = 1 h, 35-min time point) (Fluoview FV1000 confocal fluorescence microscopy) [1]

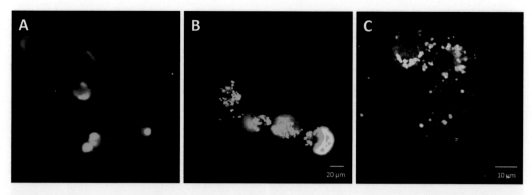

Fig. 2 Dual-color DU-145 human prostate cancer cell death induced by *S. typhimurium* A1-R. (**A**) Untreated dual-color DU-145 human prostate cancer cells (0 time point); (**B**) *S. typhimurium* A1-R-GFP invasion and proliferation in the DU-145 cells (2-h time point); (**C**) DU-145 cell death caused by bursting after extensive intracellular bacterial proliferation (24-h time point) (Fluoview FV1000 confocal fluorescence microscopy) [1]

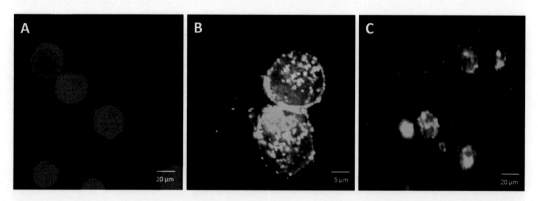

Fig. 3 LNCaP-RFP human prostate cancer cell death induced by *S. typhimurium* A1-R-GFP. (**A**) Untreated LNCaP-RFP human prostate cancer cells (0 time point); (**B**) *S. typhimurium* A1-R-GFP invasion and proliferation in the DU-145 cells (24-h time point); (**C**) LNCaP cell death caused by bursting after extensive intracellular bacterial proliferation (48-h time point) (Fluoview FV1000 confocal fluorescence microscopy) [1]

Multiphoton tomography was used to visualize *S. typhimurium* A1-R targeting the Lewis lung carcinoma (LLC) cells growing subcutaneously in nude mice. Tomography demonstrated that bacterially infected cancer cells greatly expanded and burst and thereby lost viability (Figs. 4, 5, 6 and 7) [2].

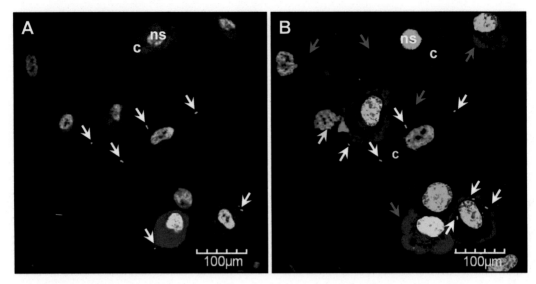

Fig. 4 In vitro imaging of dual-color Lewis lung carcinoma (LLC) cancer cells expressing GFP in the nucleus (ns) and DsRed in the cytoplasm (c) during bacteria treatment. GFP-labeled *Salmonella typhimurium* A1-R was applied to the LLC cancer cells. (**A**) 10 min after treatment with bacteria. *White arrows* show that bacteria invaded the cancer cells. (**B**) The same cancer cells were monitored 45 min after treatment with *S. typhimurium* A1-R. The cancer cells expanded, burst, and lost viability. *Blue arrows* show micro-blebs. The *yellow arrow* shows a damaged nucleus. Cells were imaged with a FU1000 confocal microscope at 473 nm for GFP excitation and 559 nm for DsRed excitation. Detection filters BA490-540 for GFP emission and BA575-675 for DsRed emission were used [2]

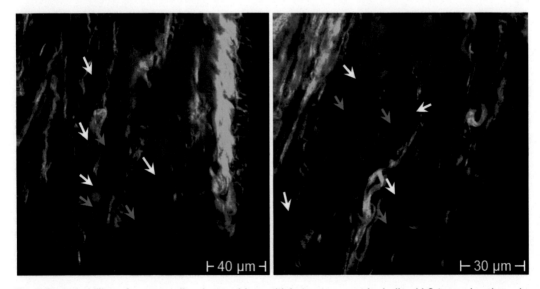

Fig. 5 Bacteria killing of cancer cells, observed by multiphoton tomography in live LLC tumor-bearing mice treated with *Salmonella typhimurium* A1-R. Extracellular matrix collagen was imaged by second-harmonic generation (SHG) without labeling (depicted in *green color*). Cancer cells expressing DsRed were visualized by two-photon excitation (*red color*). The tomographic images revealed that bacterially-infected cancer cells greatly expanded and burst and thereby lost viability similar to in vitro experiments (*see* Fig. 1). DsRed was excited at 920 nm and SHG at 790 nm. *Blue arrows* show the cell nuclei. *White arrows* show microblebs and swollen cytoplasm [2]

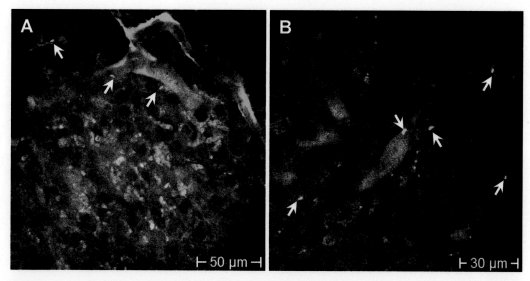

Fig. 6 In vivo multiphoton tomography with filter configuration II was used to separate GFP, DsRed, and auto-fluorescence signals. DsRed cancer cells (*red*), nestin-GFP-expressing capillaries, *S. typhimurium* A1-R-GFP bacteria, and stromal cells (autofluorescence) were imaged in live mice. (**a**) Mouse expressing nestin-GFP in capillaries was used to monitor bacteria invasion in the vessels. Single *S. typhimurium* A1-R-GFP bacteria (*white arrows*) are seen inside and outside of capillaries. (**b**) DsRed cancer cells, *S. typhimurium* A1-R-GFP bacteria, and autofluorescent stromal cells were imaged. *White arrows* demonstrate that GFP-expressing *S. typhimurium* A1-R bacteria target the DsRed cancer cells several minutes after injection of bacteria into the tail vein [2]

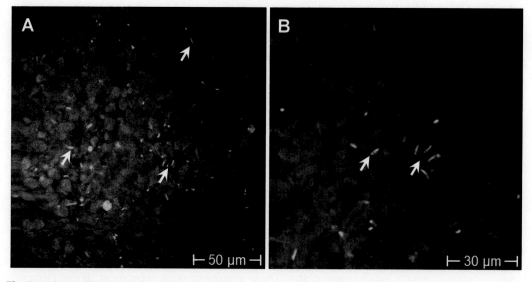

Fig. 7 In vivo multiphoton tomography imaging of an LLC tumor in a live mouse 2 days after treatment. *Blue-green-yellow* emission arises from autofluorescent stromal cells, red fluorescence from DsRed cancer cells, and bright-green fluorescence from *S. typhimurium* A1-R-GFP bacteria. Single bacteria (*white arrows*) and bacteria colonies (*red arrows*) are seen inside the tumor. Images (**a**) and (**b**) are obtained with different magnification and from different areas of the tumor [2]

2 Clinical Potential of Bacterial Therapy

A human patient who had an advanced leiomyosarcoma was treated with an intratumoral (i.t.) injection of *Clostridium novyi*-NT spores. This treatment reduced the tumor within and surrounding the bone. However, since it was used on only one of many metastases in this patient, she eventually died [3]. Systemic treatment would have more potential, but may not be possible with an obligate anaerobe. A facultative anaerobe such as *Salmonella* has more potential to treat metastatic disease as we have seen in the chapters in this book.

3 Potential Best Mode for Clinical Application of *S. typhimurium* A1-R Against Cancer

3.1 Liver Metastasis of Colon Cancer

In an orthotopic liver metastasis mouse model, *S. typhimurium* A1-R targeted liver metastases, and significantly reduced metastatic growth. The results of this study demonstrated the future clinical potential of *S. typhimurium* A1-R targeting of liver metastasis [4].

In a subsequent study, nude mice with a single liver metastasis were randomized into bright-light surgery (BLS) or BLS in combination with adjuvant treatment with tumor-targeting *S. typhimurium* A1-R. Residual tumor fluorescence after BLS was clearly visualized at high magnification by fluorescence imaging. Adjuvant treatment with *S. typhimurium* A1-R was highly effective to increase survival and disease-free survival after BLS of liver metastasis by eradicating the residual cancer cells [5].

3.2 Decoy Chemotherapy

The phase of the cell cycle can determine whether a cancer cell can respond to a given drug. As described in chapter 14 of the present volume, monitored real-time cell cycle dynamics of cancer cells throughout a live tumor intravitally using a fluorescence ubiquitination cell cycle indicator (FUCCI) before, during, and after chemotherapy. Approximately 90 % of cancer cells in the center and 80 % of total cells of an established tumor are also in G_0/G_1 phase. Approximately 75 % of cancer cells far from (>100 μm) tumor blood vessels of an established tumor are in G_0/G_1. Cytotoxic agents killed only proliferating cancer cells at the surface, or near blood vessels, and, in contrast, had little effect on quiescent cancer cells, which are the vast majority of an established tumor. Moreover, resistant quiescent cancer cells restarted cycling after the cessation of chemotherapy. These results suggest why most drugs currently in clinical use, which target cancer cells in $S/G_2/M$, are mostly ineffective on solid tumors. However, when the tumors were treated with S. typhimurium A1-R, the quiescent cells were decoyed to cycle and were readily killed by chemotherapy. This type of treatment is called decoy chemotherapy [6, 7].

3.3 Combination of S. typhimurium A1-R and Anti-angiogenesis Therapy

The efficacy of tumor-targeting *Salmonella typhimurium* A1-R treatment following anti-vascular endothelial growth factor (VEGF) therapy on VEGF-positive human pancreatic cancer was tested. A pancreatic cancer patient-derived orthotopic xenograft (PDOX) that was VEGF positive and an orthotopic VEGF-positive human pancreatic cancer cell line (MiaPaCa-2-GFP) as well as a VEGF-negative pancreatic cancer cell line (Panc-1) were tested. Nude mice with these tumors were treated with gemcitabine (GEM), bevacizumab (BEV), and *S. typhimurium* A1-R. BEV/GEM followed by *S. typhimurium* A1-R significantly reduced tumor weight compared to BEV/GEM treatment alone in the PDOX and MiaPaCa-2 models. Neither treatment was as effective in the Panc-1 VEGF-negative model as in the VEGF-positive models. These results demonstrate that *S. typhimurium* A1-R following anti-angiogenic therapy is effective on pancreatic cancer including the PDOX model, suggesting clinical potential [8].

3.4 Cancer Stem Cell Therapy with the Combination of S. typhimurium A1-R and Chemotherapy

The XPA-1 human pancreatic cancer cell line is dimorphic, with spindle stem-like cells and round non-stem cells. IC_{50} values for 5-fluorouracil (5-FU) or cisplatinum (CDDP) of stem-like XPA-1 cells were significantly higher than those of non-stem XPA-1 cells. In contrast, there was no difference between the efficacy of *S. typhimurium* A1-R on stem-like and non-stem XPA-1 cells. In vivo, 5-FU and *S. typhimurium* A1-R significantly reduced the tumor weight of non-stem XPA-1 cells. In contrast, only *S. typhimurium* A1-R significantly reduced tumor weight of stem-like XPA-1 cells. The combination of *S. typhimurium* A1-R with 5-FU improved the antitumor efficacy compared with 5-FU monotherapy on the stem-like cells. These results indicate that *S. typhimurium* A1-R is a promising therapy for chemoresistant pancreatic cancer stem-like cells [9].

References

1. Uchugonova A, Zhang Y, Salz R, Liu F, Suetsugu A, Zhang L et al (2015) Imaging the different mechanisms of prostate cancer-cell killing by tumor-targeting *Salmonella typhimurium* A1-R. Anticancer Res 35:5225–5229

2. Uchugonova A, Zhao M, Zhang Y, Weinigel M, König K, Hoffman RM (2012) Cancer-cell killing by engineered *Salmonella* imaged by multiphoton tomography in live mice. Anticancer Res 32:4331–4338

3. Roberts NJ, Zhang L, Janku F, Collins A, Bai RY, Staedtke V et al (2014) Intratumoral injection of Clostridium novyi-NT spores induces antitumor responses. Sci Transl Med 6:249ra111

4. Murakami T, Hiroshima Y, Zhao M, Zhang Y, Chishima T, Tanaka K et al (2015) Thera peutic efficacy of tumor-targeting Salmonella typhimurium A1-R on human colorectal cancer liver metastasis in orthotopic nude-mouse models. Oncotarget 6:31368–31377

5. Murakami T, Hiroshima Y, Zhao M, Zhang Y, Chishima T, Tanaka K et al (2015) Adjuvant treatment with tumor-targeting *Salmonella typhimurium* A1-R reduces recurrence and increases survival after liver metastasis resection

in an orthotopic nude mouse model. Oncotarget 6:41856–41862

6. Yano S, Zhang Y, Miwa S, Tome Y, Hiroshima Y, Uehara F et al (2014) Spatial-temporal FUCCI imaging of each cell in a tumor demonstrates locational dependence of cell cycle dynamics and chemoresponsiveness. Cell Cycle 13:2110–2119

7. Yano S, Zhang Y, Zhao M, Hiroshima Y, Miwa S, Uehara F et al (2014) Tumor-targeting Salmonella typhimurium A1-R decoys quiescent cancer cells to cycle as visualized by FUCCI imaging and become sensitive to chemotherapy. Cell Cycle 13:3958–3963.

8. Hiroshima Y, Zhang Y, Murakami T, Maawy AA, Miwa S, Yamamoto M et al (2014) Efficacy of tumor-targeting *Salmonella typhimurium* A1-R in combination with anti-angiogenesis therapy on a pancreatic cancer patient-derived orthotopic xenograph (PDOX) and cell line mouse models. Oncotarget 5:12346–12357

9. Hiroshima Y, Zhao M, Zhang Y, Maawy A, Hassanein MK, Uehara F et al (2013) Comparison of efficacy of *Salmonella typhimurium* A1-R and chemotherapy on stem-like and non-stem human pancreatic cancer cells. Cell Cycle 12:2774–2780

INDEX

Robert M. Hoffman (ed.), *Bacterial Therapy of Cancer: Methods and Protocols*, Methods in Molecular Biology, vol. 1409,
DOI 10.1007/978-1-4939-3515-4, © Springer Science+Business Media New York 2016

Printed in the United States
By Bookmasters